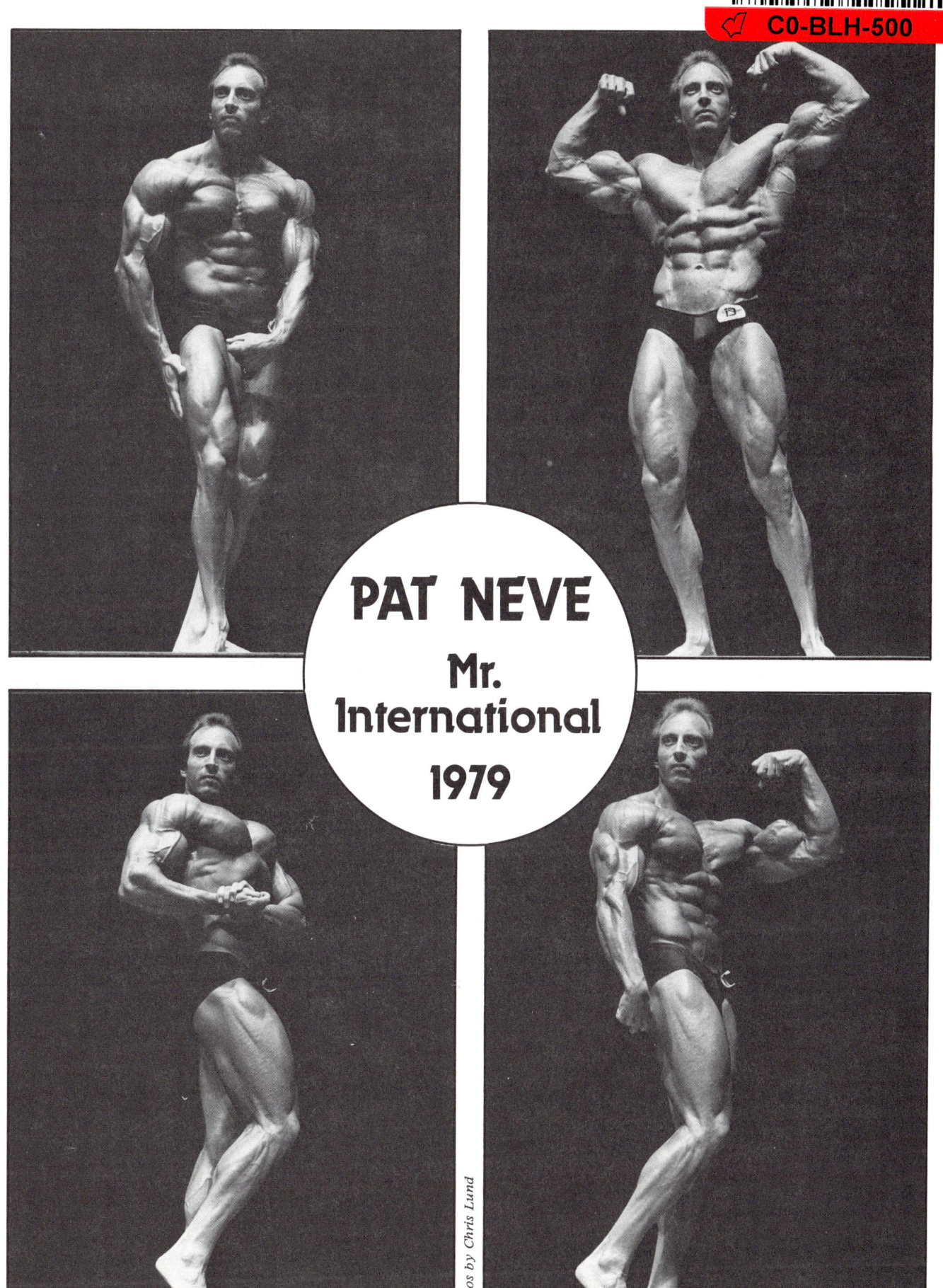

PAT NEVE'S BODYBUILDING DIET BOOK

By
Vicki Neve

A Self-Fulfillment Book

ISBN: 0-914778-33-1

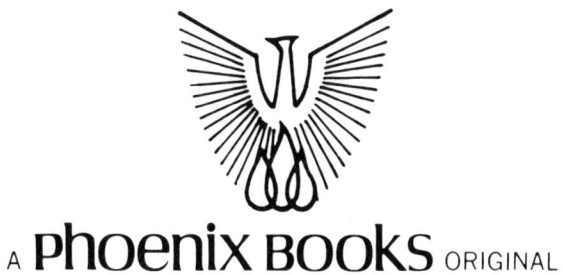

A PHOENIX BOOKS ORIGINAL

PHOENIX BOOKS/PUBLISHERS
Phoenix, Arizona U.S.A.

Dedication

This book is dedicated to my husband, the truest athlete I've ever known. His self-discipline, determination and dedication to the sport of bodybuilding has inspired me beyond words. His example has instilled in me an overwhelming respect for all who relentlessly test their endurance and abilities to reach physical excellence.

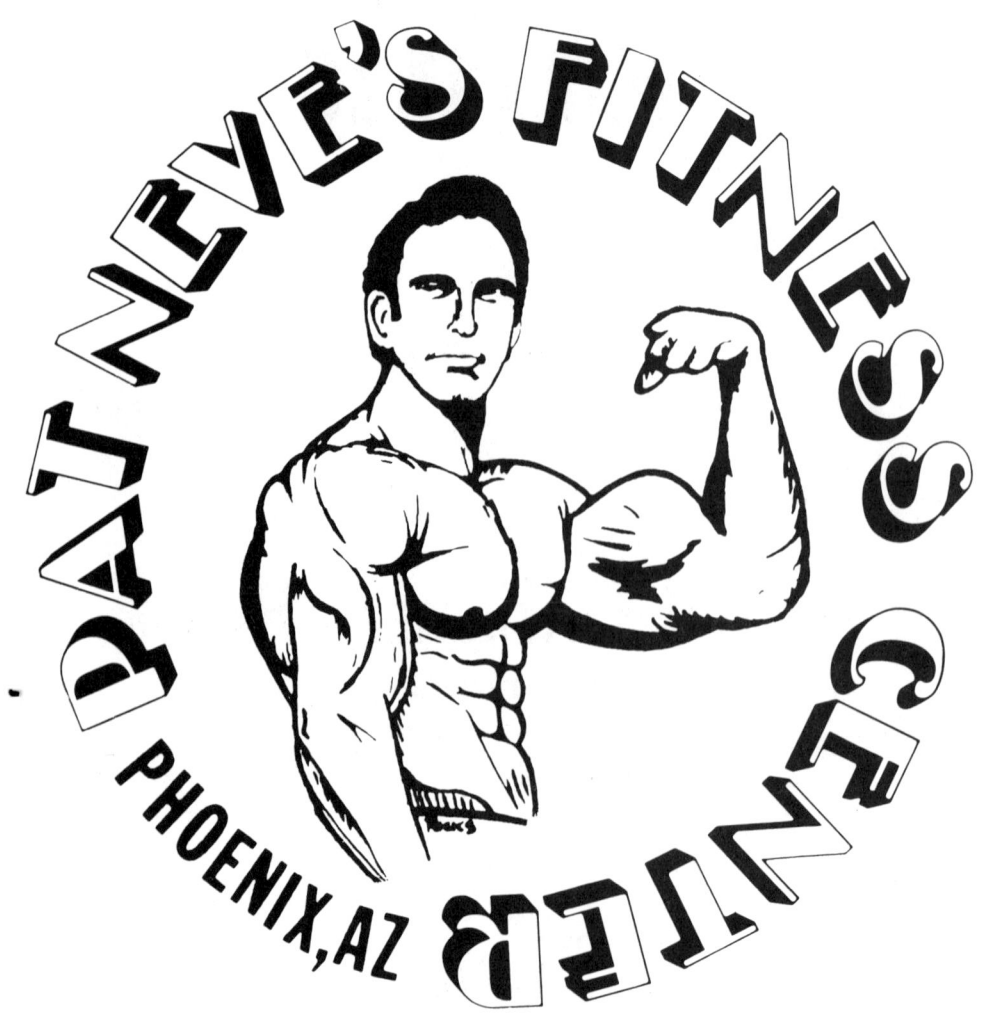

Published by Phoenix Books/Publishers, P.O. Box 32008, Phoenix, AZ. 85064 USA. Copyright (C) 1981 by Vicki Neve. All rights reserved. No part of this material may be reproduced in any form by any means without written permission from the publisher. Manufactured in the United States of America.

ISBN: 0-914778-33-1

About the Author

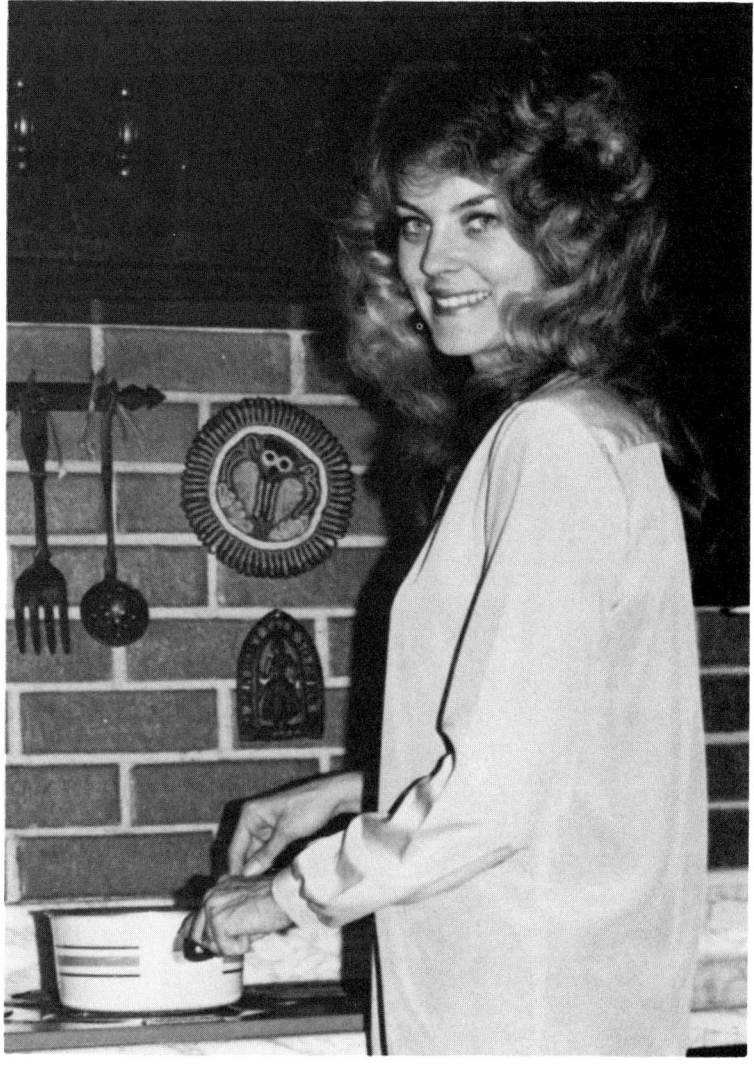

ABOUT THE AUTHOR (By the Author)... Pat and I met in 1966, just weeks after he had placed 2nd in his first physique contest. During the 5-year engagement that followed, a whole new world opened up for me. I was introduced to bodybuilding. Phrases like bulking-up, cutting-up and pumping-up became commonplace to me. Because I loved the man, I began to love his sport.

In those early years the competition wasn't very tough. The winner was usually obvious the moment he stepped onto the posing platform. But as the sport grew, so did the competition. By the time we were married in 1971 bodybuilding had become established as a major sport and was turning out hundreds of great physiques.

Pat and I grew along with bodybuilding, and soon realized that pumping iron just wasn't enough anymore. We started concentrating more on nutrition and food preparation. I developed diets and recipes which Pat applied to his training. After each contest we analyzed the diet techniques until ultimately we developed the *Countdown Diet* which helped make Pat a champion in bodybuilding.

Contents

I
WHY A DIET BOOK FOR BODYBUILDERS?.. 7

II
BODYBUILDING: THE SPORT... 9
    Making It As A Professional 10
    The Competition... 10

III
A DIET GUIDE TO BODYBUILDING.. 14
    Muscle And Joint Pain.. 14
    Carbohydrates And The Bodybuilder 14
    Steroids And The Bodybuilder 15
    Meat And The Bodybuilder... 16
    Fats And The Bodybuilder 16
    The Egg And Cholesterol... 17
    Eating On The Road 17
    What About Sugar?.. 18
    Bodybuilding Supplements... 18
    Natural Vitamins Vs. Synthetic... 19
    Food Concentrates 19
    Diuretics And The Bodybuilder... 19
    Vascularity 19

IV
14-DAY WEIGHT-LOSS DIET AND MENUS... 21

V
14-DAY WEIGHT-GAIN DIET AND MENUS... 27

VI
PAT'S FAMOUS COUNTDOWN DIET... 34

VII
WOMEN'S BODYBUILDING AND 14-DAY MENU PLAN 43

VIII
THE LOW CARBOHYDRATE DIET COOKBOOK 51

IX
ATHLETE'S VITAMIN AND MINERAL GUIDE... 66

X
A FOOD GUIDE FOR BODYBUILDING... 70

I
WHY A DIET BOOK FOR BODYBUILDERS?

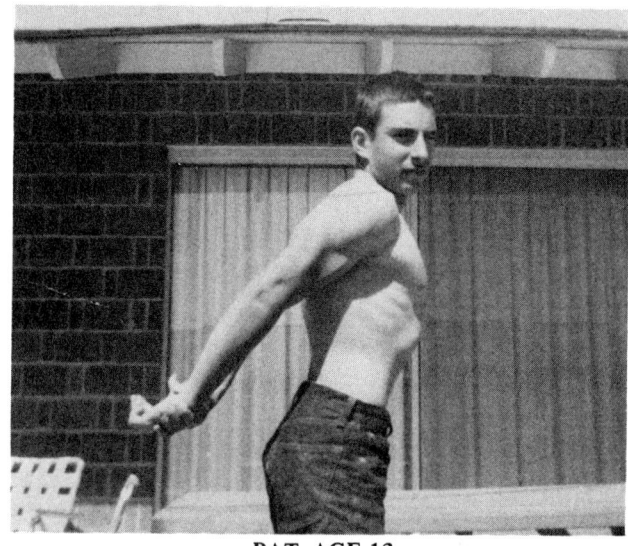
PAT, AGE 13

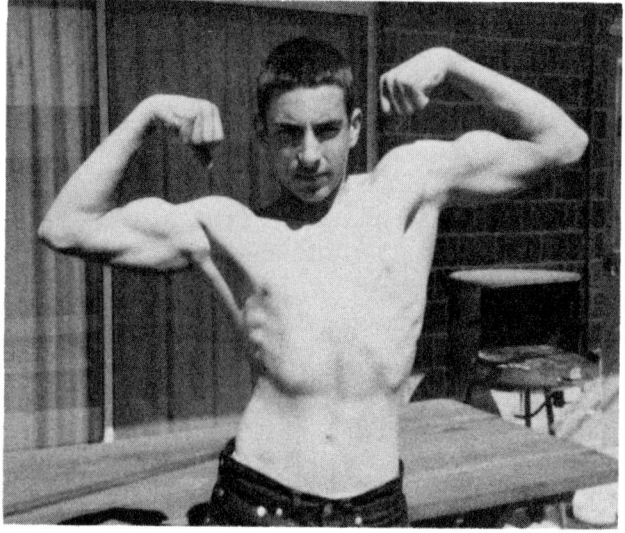

Countless numbers of books have been written on diets. Different approaches to different methods have been designed for gaining and losing weight. This is yet another approach to diet through specific techniques developed and tested by a family dramatically dedicated to body fitness.

While training for a career in bodybuilding my husband, Pat Neve, and I have experimented with literally thousands of diets to achieve the total "peak" in his body's condition. For over 12 years we have worked at finding a sound combination in diet, weight training and vitamin supplements needed to compete in the sport of bodybuilding. We perfected various diets needed in Pat's training for weight loss, weight gain, maintaining weight and finally the intense countdown diet used for six weeks before a competition.

After opening our own health club, we were able to apply these diets to other individuals' training programs. Outstanding results were obtained by those we counciled in bodybuilding as well as in other sports such as football, track, wrestling and gymnastics.

We further explored our diet techniques on our members who just wanted to get in good physical condition and maintain it. This group included housewives, mothers, businessmen and active career women, who for one reason or another had fallen below their physical standard of condition. The results were overwhelming. Many members came to our health facility expecting to exercise away their unwanted flab, and to condition their physique while still eating anything they wanted, and were surprised at the emphasis we placed on diet. Pat and I feel diet is 75 percent of the program.

Each metabolism is unique in its performance and its ability to process set rules of a diet, so flexibility is a very important factor. Each of our members are put on one of three diet techniques. Then after each week of following the prescribed diet and exercise program, the results are weighed. Not only do we check for pounds lost or gained, but also the person's level of energy while on the diet and overall muscle tone developed through the exercise and weight training program.

Then if necessary adjustments are made in the individual diet and exercise program to best suit that person's needs. For instance, while on a weight loss diet of low carbohydrates the body's energy level often suffers. If too much fatigue causes a problem an extra five grams of carbohydrates a day will often meet these energy needs and still produce a satisfactory weight loss. Again, a key factor is being able to judge how your body reacts to each diet, and being flexible.

These diet techniques are not secret. Actually, they are fundamental in what we have learned over the past 20 years about carbohydrates.

We went back to some basic theories and worked at setting up complete menus and interesting recipes to make the individual diet more flexible. Our 12 years of experience has proven instrumental in Pat's achievements in both Power Lifting and bodybuilding competitions. His record speaks for itself.

- 1967 Mr. Phoenix
- 1968 Mr. Arizona
- 1969 Mr. Southwest
- 1970 Arizona State Power Lifting Champion, 181 pound class
- 1971 Mr. Valley of the Sun
- 1972 Mr. Western America
- 1973 Jr. Mr. USA Runner-up
- 1974 Mr. USA & Mr. Southwest USA
- 1975 Mr. America, Class I
- 1976 Mr. America, Class I
- 1977 PBA Pro Mr. Universe, First Runner-up
- 1978 WBBG Pro Mr. World, First Runner-up
- 1979 U.S. Representative in the Mr. Universe Competition
- 1979 Pro Mr. International Middle-Weight Class

From 1971 through 1974, Pat was the World Record Holder in the Bench Press, 181-Pound Class.

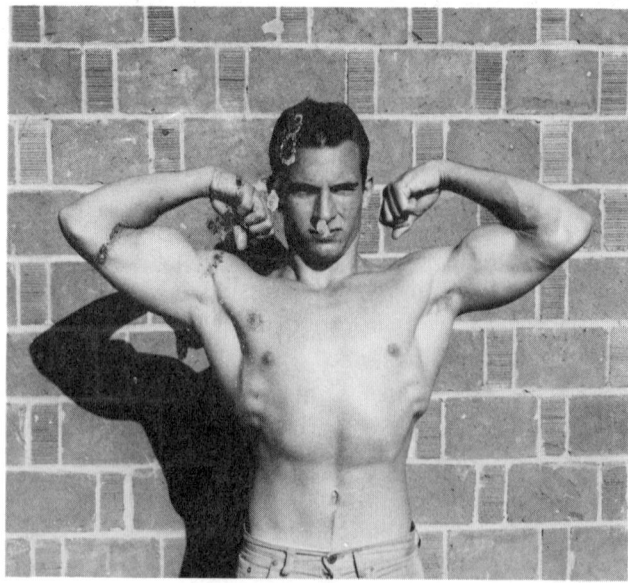

PAT, AGE 15

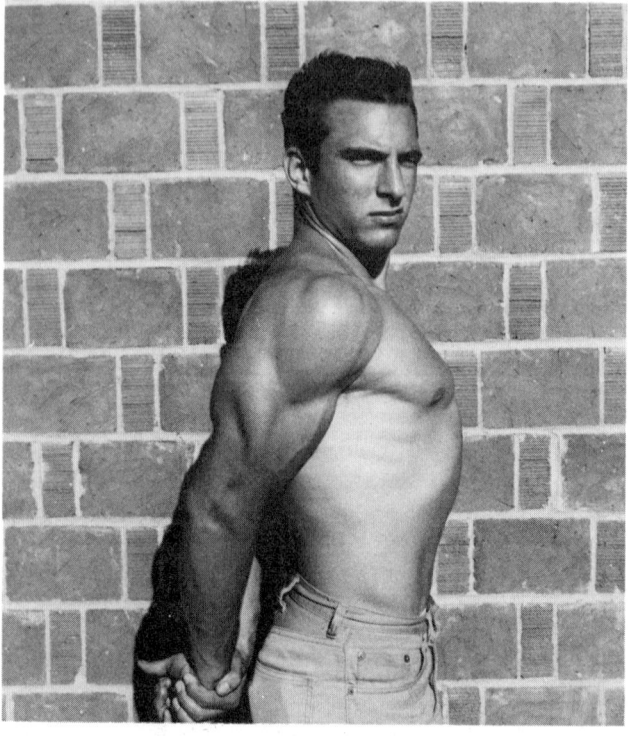

II

BODYBUILDING: THE SPORT

𝓑odybuilding! Some call it a show, comparing it to a female beauty contest. Others prefer to call it an art. The bodybuilders themselves vehemently call it a sport, and justifiably so.

The degree of training, dedication and self-discipline that goes into bodybuilding surpasses the requirements of any other commonly practiced sport in the world. The number of athletes training for bodybuilding today has reached record highs. This has come about, in part, because of the increased exposure bodybuilding has received in recent years. The quantity and quality of competition has also improved tremendously.

Though considered a new sport, bodybuilding goes back many years. The first Mr. America contest was held in 1938. The youngest Mr. America was 19, the oldest was 37.

Today, competitive bodybuilding is divided into two areas of competition: the AAU (Amateur Athletic Union), and Professional. The AAU organizes various state meets for the beginning bodybuilder. If a bodybuilder is to continue his career in the sport he must first win his state title. This entitles him to enter the Jr. Mr. USA, Sr. Mr. USA, Jr. Mr. America, and finally one of the most prestigious titles in bodybuilding, the AAU Mr. America title.

Many bodybuilders are lured away from the AAU to professional competition long before winning the Mr. America crown. There are usually two reasons for this: the financial opportunities or because they have been disappointed by judging decisions. Although this move prohibits them from entering any further AAU competition, some feel the exchange is well worth the sacrifice.

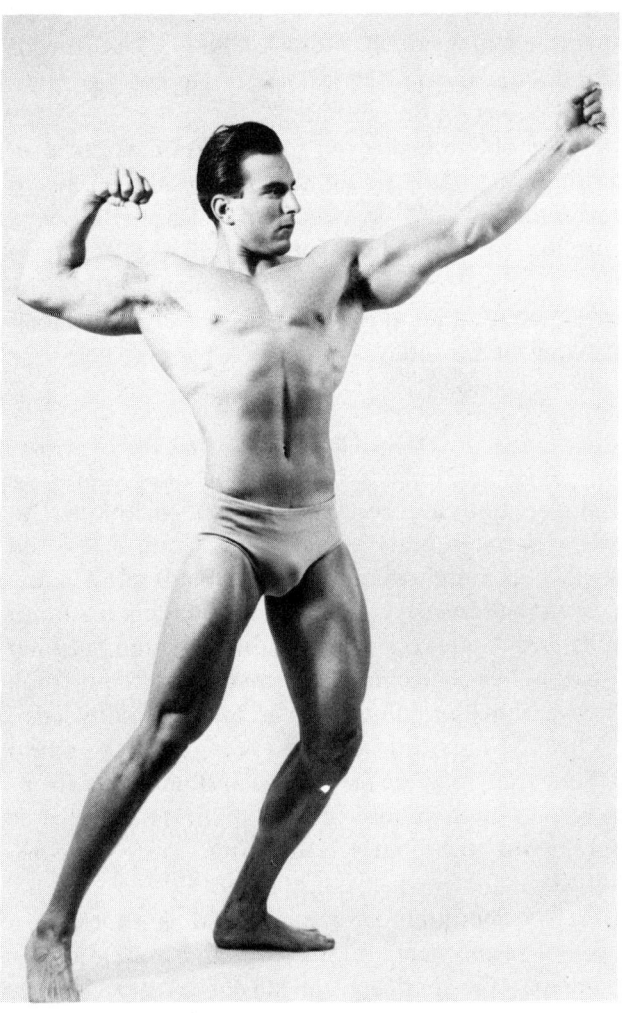

PAT, 18, TRAINING FOR MR. ARIZONA CONTEST

MAKING IT AS A PROFESSIONAL

If a bodybuilder is good enough to make it in the professional ranks it can be very rewarding. There are various requests for paid exhibitions (invitations to guest-pose at contests around the country) and seminars (discussions on individual training techniques and bodybuilding theories). Also there are opportunities for product endorsements.

As a professional there are also opportunities outside the sport of bodybuilding. Some bodybuilders have gone on to do television commericals and movies. Two outstanding examples whom bodybuilding takes great pride in are Lou Ferrigno (Pro Mr. America; Mr. Universe) and Arnold Schwarzenegger, seven-time winner of the famed Mr. Olympia contest. Lou made an impressive appearance on the Super Stars and co-stars in the television series, *The Hulk*. Arnold was acclaimed for his contributions to the book *Pumping Iron* and was winner of the Golden Globe Award for his part in the movie *Stay Hungry*. He has also published books on bodybuilding.

Arnold remains a key instrument in promoting an awareness on the part of the public to bodybuilding, and provides rare insights into bodybuilding, the art and the sport.

Thanks to the dedication of many within the sport, bodybuilding has become one of the fastest growing sports today.

THE COMPETITION

Bodybuilding today has become almost a science, applying several different techniques to reach perfection in a body's physique. The old myth that muscle men are muscleheads has become a thing of the past. Many bodybuilders maintain substantial careers outside of bodybuilding in such areas as law, teaching and medicine. One thing they all have in common is an in-depth knowledge of health, nutrition and kinesiology, or the study of the principles of mechanics and anatomy in relation to human movement. This knowledge is applied to the intense training necessary for competition.

The bodybuilder's main goal is to reach a "peak" in physical conditioning and muscle development. Competitors are judged on muscle size, symmetry, muscle definition and presentation. While training for competition certain techniques are applied to the training program in the areas of weight training, diet and vitamin supplements. There is an extra concentration placed on skin tone and skin color. Last, but by no means least, each bodybuilder takes on the study and continuous practice of physique presentation in the form of a posing routine — next to diet, probably the most important area of competition conditioning.

After months of rigorous weight training, time-tabled diet techniques, hours of sunbathing and skin conditioning, each bodybuilder is given about three minutes to present their physique to the judges. Knowing how to present each muscle group to his best advantage is in a bodybuilder's posing ability — and lack of it can lose him the title.

Sometimes in the area of presentation we find a mysterious quality called charisma. The vibrant personality, total awareness and confidence in one's own ability. The great Arnold Schwarzenegger had it as does Frank Zane, three-time winner of the Mr. Olympia contest.

Although some feel you either have charisma or you don't, I believe a certain amount of it can be developed through the knowledge and confidence gained in one's own training techniques.

With this purpose in mind, I would like to share the diet and supplement techniques used in Pat Neve's training program — techniques that have proven effective in Pat's own career in bodybuilding.

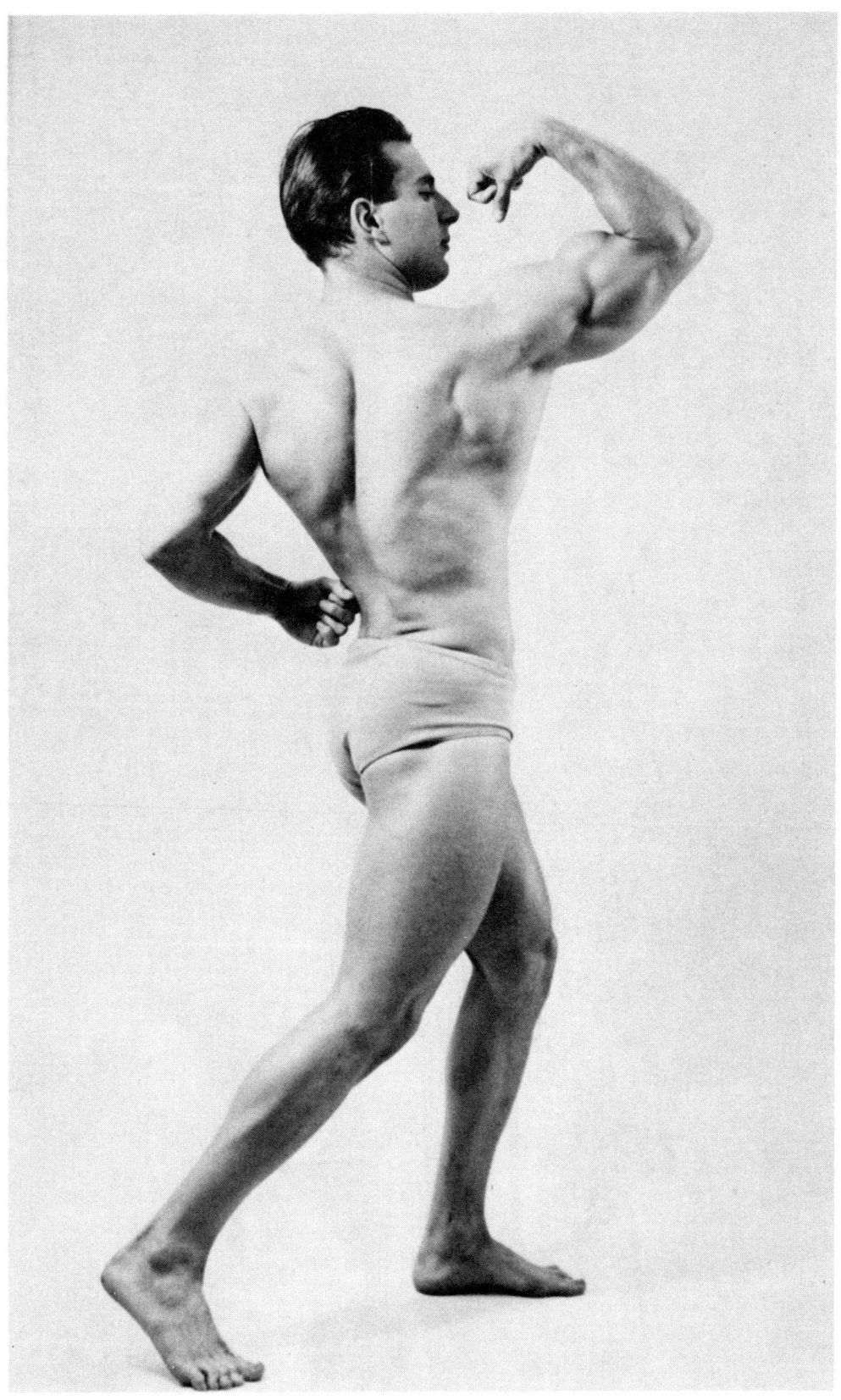

PAT, 18, TRAINING FOR MR. ARIZONA CONTEST

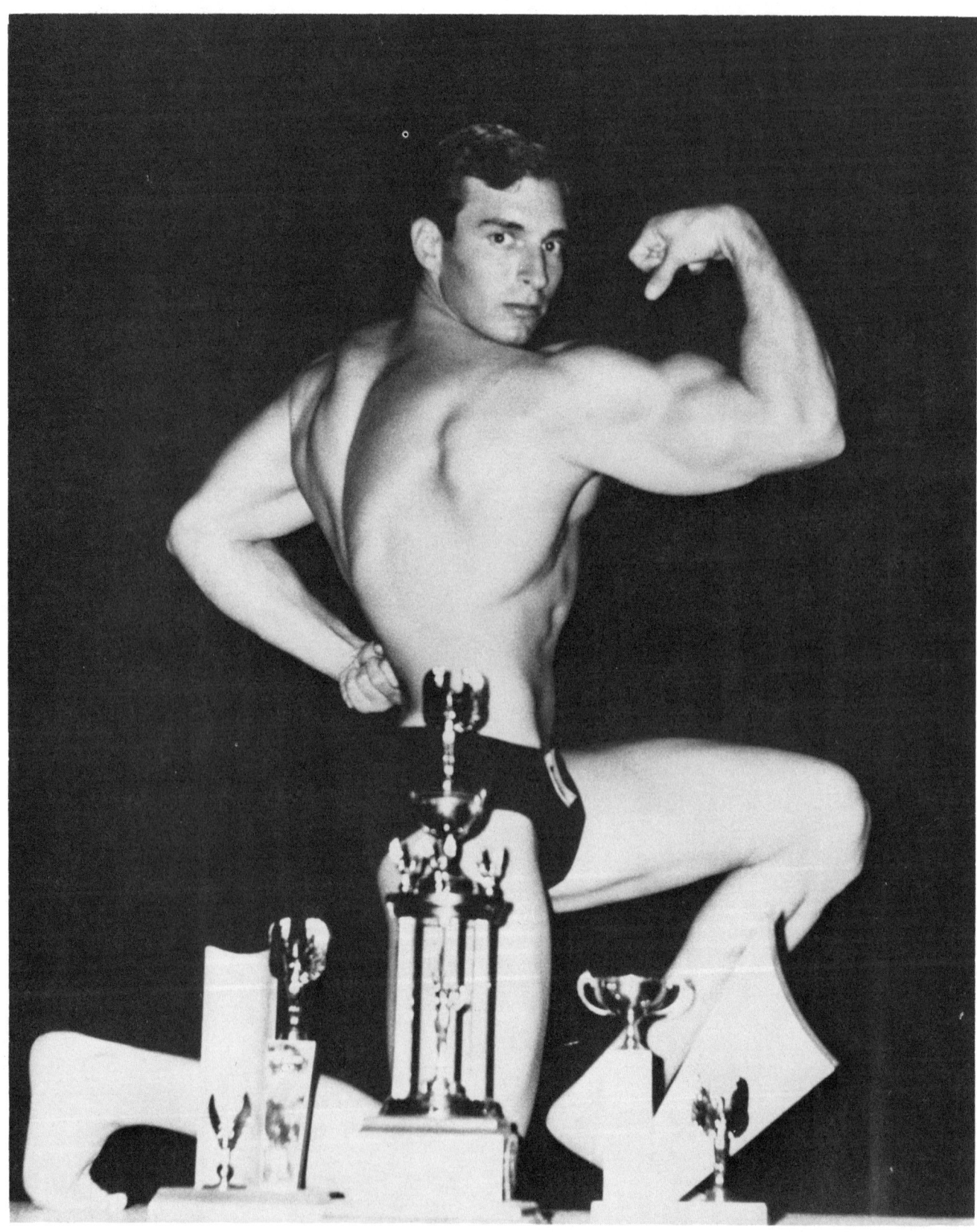

PAT, 19, WINNING THE MR. ARIZONA CONTEST

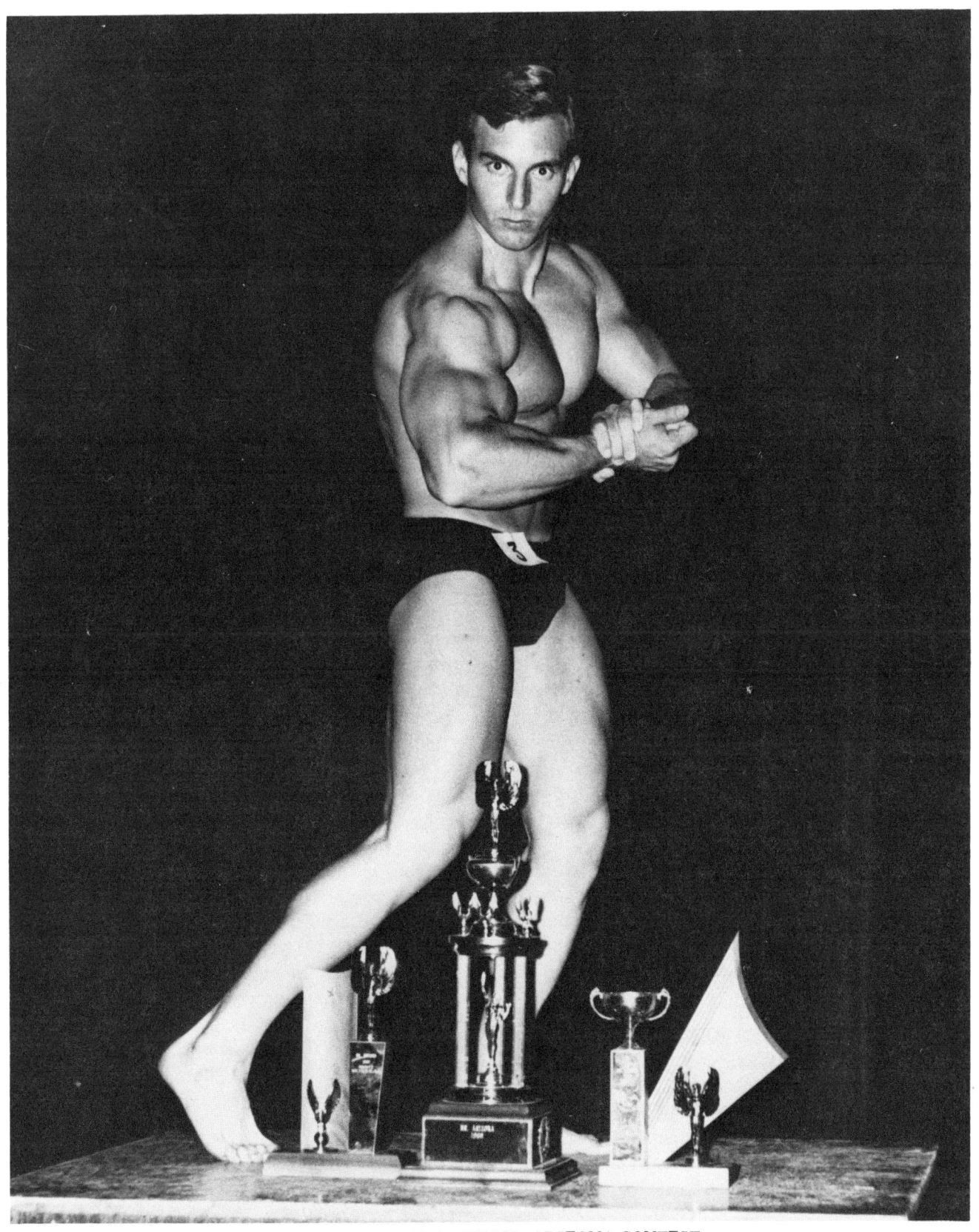

PAT, 19, WINNING THE MR. ARIZONA CONTEST

III

A DIET GUIDE TO BODYBUILDING

As a bodybuilder's wife I am continually asked about diet and its application to contest training. Often I feel the younger bodybuilders are trying to catch me off-guard in the hope that I will slip and give out some secret to diet or training in bodybuilding.

There are no secrets! Self-discipline, determination and a sound knowledge of the human body and its nutritional needs are the bodybuilder's tools to success.

There is one thing I am totally convinced of. There is no **one** perfect formula designed for all bodybuilders. Too many great physiques claim too many different techniques in training. The obvious conclusion is finding a particular formula that works for you — usually through trial and error.

However, there are some basic nutritional facts that can be shared to benefit everyone training for bodybuilding (or any other kind of athletic sport). The following is a collection of topics I have most often been asked about in relation to bodybuilding.

MUSCLE AND JOINT PAIN

This is probably one of the biggest complaints among bodybuilders, and deservedly so. The first thing to consider is the tremendous strain placed on both muscles and joints during hard contest training. To some extent the pain should be expected and accepted as part of the sport. Many bodybuilders actually like the muscle soreness as an indication of muscle growth.

But should a particular ache or pain persist to the point of hindering the workout, there are three things to consider. First it might be an actual injury to the muscle, joint or even the tendons and ligaments. In this case you would be wise to discontinue the exercise causing pain in the particular area. Don't push an injury, or you may cause serious permanent damage. There is usually more than one exercise designed to work each muscle group. Try an alternative until the injury is healed. Also ice the area until completely numb and apply a gentle massage. This should heal a minor injury in about a week.

The second thing to consider is that aching muscles and joints often indicate a calcium deficiency. This is easily possible during training months when dairy products are limited. An increase in calcium supplements might prove beneficial.

If all else fails, a third area to explore is your uric acid level. Have it checked by a physician. Uric acid is a factor in gout and can cause extreme joint pain. One disadvantage to a high protein diet abundant in meat is a rise in uric acid. A natural aid for this is black cherry concentrate, sold in health food stores. There is also medication for treating it; should you confirm its presence.

CARBOHYDRATES AND THE BODYBUILDER

Carbohydrates are essential to the human diet. A bodybuilder needs the energy supplied by carbohydrates more than the average person. So why do so many bodybuilders choose low carbohydrate diets? As discussed earlier, it is the **kind** of carbohydrates that are important and the overeating of a good thing that is discouraged.

A bodybuilder should limit his carbohydrate intake to complex or unrefined carbohydrates such as raw fruits and vegetables. If you must cook them, cook them as little as possible.

During contest training the idea is to supply only the energy needs for training without adding extra body fat. Some good choices would be cantaloupe, strawberries, peaches, green beans, broccoli, and zucchini. Fruit and vegetable juices contain twice — some times three times — the amount of calories as in the single whole raw fruit or vegetable they represent. Do not drink them while training. They can smooth you out.

As competition draws nearer even low carbohydrate fruits should be eliminated because of the fruit sugar they contain. About the last two weeks before a contest you would be wise to rely on low carbohydrate vegetables for training energy. Green vegetables burn slow and provide sustained energy for the training.

Refined sugar and flour are out (see more about sugar further on!) Also be aware of refined sugar additives hiding under such aliases as sucrose, lactose, corn syrup, dextrose and corn sugar. Avoid processed foods whenever possible. They play havoc with the blood sugar levels and deplete the quality of energy.

Alcohol is another thing to avoid. It interferes with the vitamin balance and quite evidently hinders definition. It also has little if any nutritional value, which after all is the name of the game in body fitness.

STEROIDS AND THE BODYBUILDER

Steroids are growth hormones, and in extreme application, can halt the body's own natural production of these hormones. The prolonged use of steroids can cause sterility, calcium deficiencies, and even possible liver damage.

It's no secret that many pros take steroids, but by introducing steroids too early in your bodybuilding career, you are robbing your body of its natural potential. Personally, I feel the use of steroids shortens your career by shortening your natural gains.

Yet in order to face this issue realistically,

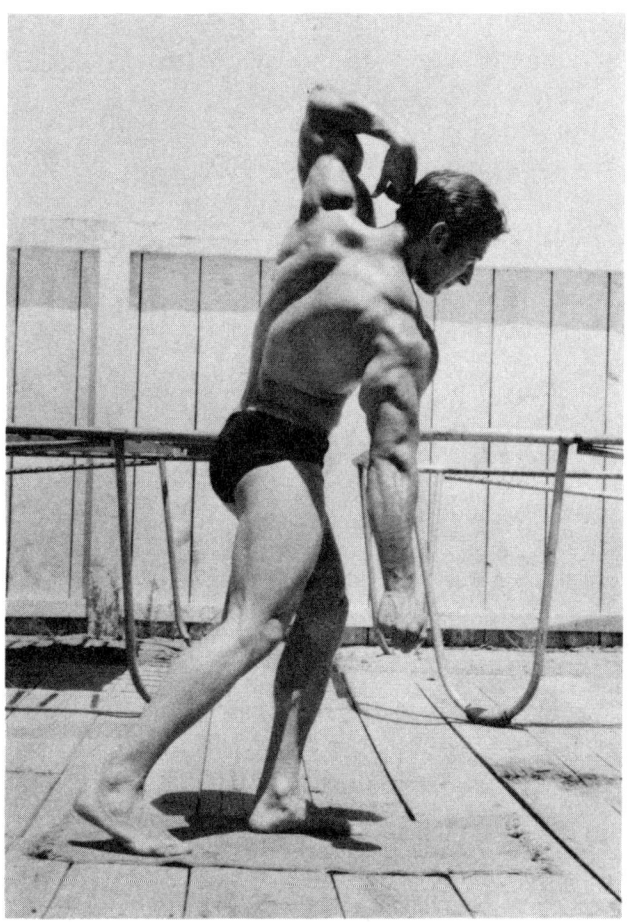

PAT, 22, TRAINING AT JERRY DOYLE'S HEALTH CLUB

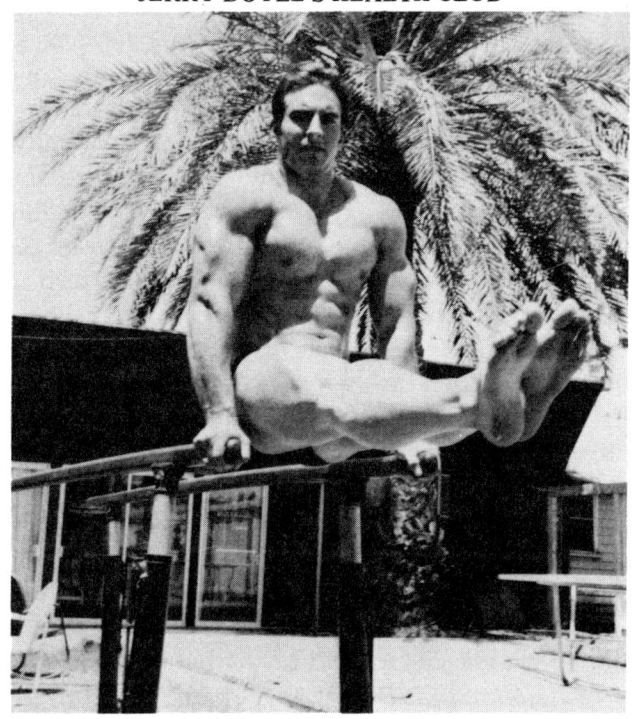

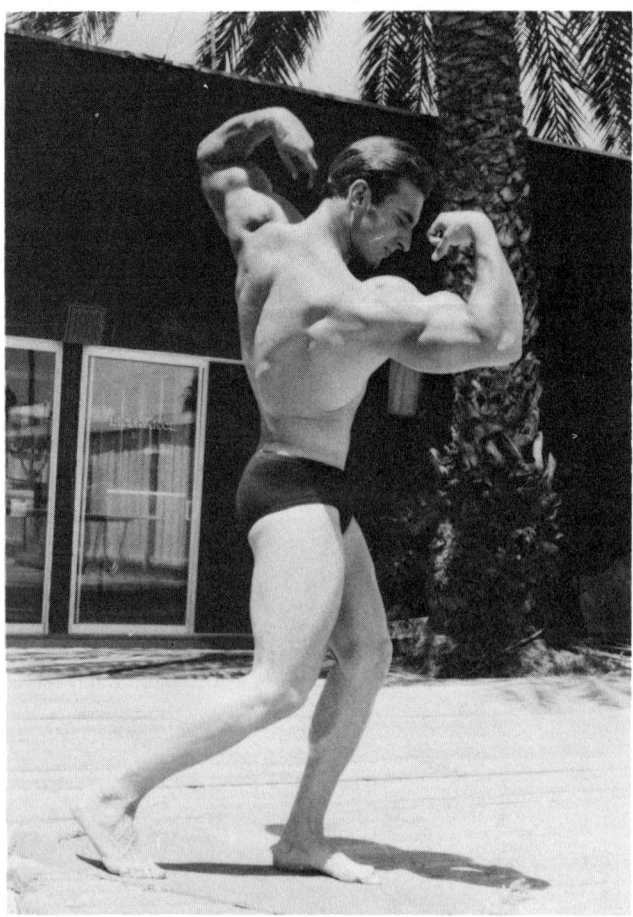

**PAT, 22, TRAINING AT
JERRY DOYLE'S HEALTH CLUB**

we have to accept the existence of steroids in bodybuilding today, then set priorities concerning their use. The practical purpose of steroids on a professional level is simple. The professional bodybuilder has already gained the muscular size and physique necessary for advanced bodybuilding competition **without** steroids, through years of hard, disciplined training. Then many pros turn to steroids to **retain** that size through excruciating contest training. This degree of training is often only a fraction away from over-training, which can lead to retarded growth and some degree of atrophy to the muscle.

But this degree of training, incorporated with intense diet techniques, establishes a warranted reason to use steroids to retain size, not build it.

If you are looking for steroids to be your short-cut to muscle growth, you might as will quit bodybuilding. You don't have what it takes to be a champion.

MEAT AND THE BODYBUILDER

There is a variety of different opinions on meat and its importance in bodybuilding. Most of what I've read on the various training programs of individual bodybuilders is acceptable. What it comes down to is what works well for you and your own food preferences. What I refer to in this book is "Pat Neve's Diet Program" and what 12 years of experimentation has proven to be effective for his physique.

Out of eight essential amino acids that the body supposedly does not manufacture, meat contains all eight! Remember, beef, lamb and pork are high in fat; while fish and fowl are lower in calories. For contest purposes, any red meat should be eaten early in the day, serving the strenuous energy needs, yet leaving time for burning up the excess fat content. As the contest draws nearer, say when it is two weeks away, it is advisable to eliminate beef, lamb and pork completely.

Fish and fowl are most acceptable during the last two weeks of training because of their lower calories and the high protein value. Another good point in meat preparation is to cook it as little as possible, or just until done. Over cooking any food robs it of many valuable vitamins and minerals. The less you cook meat the more protein you get from it.

Another factor in meat training is the acid involved. Meat, poultry and fish are acidic. Dairy products are alkaline. Although in my Bodybuilding Countdown Training Diet dairy products are discouraged, cheese is the one exception. It has the least milk sugar, and while one is training on a meat diet, will provide a good balance for the acid.

FATS AND THE BODYBUILDER

You need fats, both saturated and unsaturated. While on a low carbohydrate diet, fats help keep you satisfied, reducing your desire for sweets, and even aid in preventing the build-up of body fat from too many carbohydrates. Yet for contest training, a bodybuilder needs to limit his fats to some degree. Again, they can smooth you out and hinder maximum cuts. Fried foods are out!

The link between polyunsaturated fats and

accelerated aging is something to think about; especially in bodybuilding where maximum skin tone and texture are important.

THE EGG AND CHOLESTEROL

The poor egg came under heavy fire during the 1970's as a result of the cholesterol scare. Because of the amount of eggs used in Pat's training diet, we researched the subject of cholesterol, reading every professional opinion we could find on it. Through our studies we formed a solid belief in the egg and its nutritional value. The egg is one of our most complete foods, containing many essential nutrients in just the right proportions. The egg is an excellent source of protein yet low in carbohydrates.

As for cholesterol, many prominent nutritionists and biochemists now agree that dietary cholesterol has little effect on cholesterol levels in the blood. Further studies have revealed the importance of lowering your carbohydrate intake and exercise in reducing blood cholesterol and its related problems. During our research on cholesterol we also learned that most margarines are more saturated than butter and contain less Vitamin E and other food factors important to proper nutrition.

My basic belief on overall nutrition is moderation. In our attempts to reduce carbohydrates, we do not eliminate them completely. We simply feel the average consumption is too high. I think time will prove moderation is the key to better health, better nutrition and better bodybuilding.

ON THE ROAD

Many athletes find it difficult to eat properly while traveling to various competitions. When Pat travels to compete, I try to pack as much as I can for him to snack on. Things like hard boiled eggs, tuna salad, and raw vegetables like celery, zucchini, broccoli and cucumbers keep well in a jar or covered container with some cold water. I always pack some fruit and unsalted nuts, raisins, etc. for last-minute contest preparations. With the sometimes hectic schedules of the pre-judging, Pat relies heavily on these snacks.

Despite our efforts and because of the limited travel space, Pat is usually forced to dine out at least once. Here are some things he looks for on the restaurant menus:

Omelettes
Tuna or chicken salad
Low calorie plates
Baked fish or chicken
Dinner salad with vinegar & oil dressing
Any of the low carbohydrate vegetables
Iced tea or Perrier water

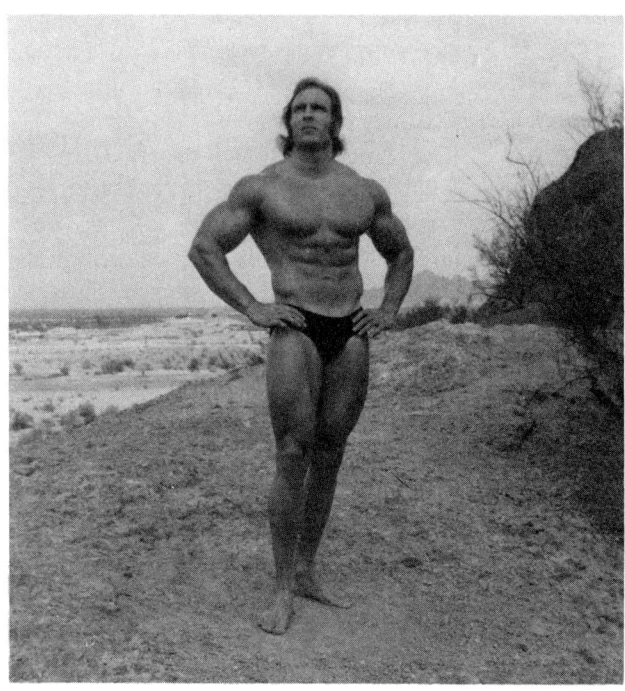

PAT, 24, TRAINING FOR MR. USA

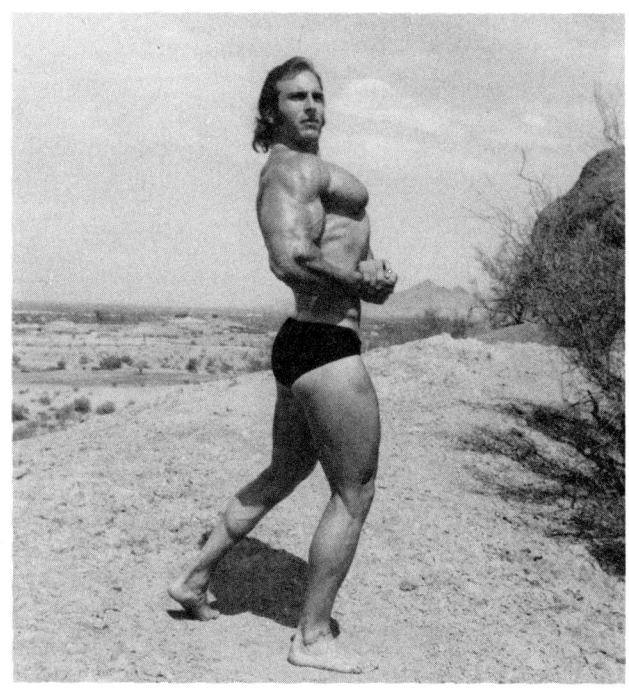

WHAT ABOUT SUGAR?

First you should understand how sugar is handled by the body. Sucrose, or white refined sugar, is absorbed from the intestine, goes through the liver and into the blood stream to be carried to all the body tissues. Any sugar which is not immediately used by the body tissues is taken from the blood, changed into fat, and stored in the body as fatty tissue.

Much of the white sugar we eat is thus rushed into the bloodstream in far greater amounts than we need, and is turned into fat.

On the other hand, natural sugars such as glucose and fructose stop when they reach the liver, and are drawn up by the blood only as they are needed. Natural sugars therefore have a much better chance of being used as energy instead of being stored as fat.

There are many types of sweeteners such as white sugar, brown sugar, molasses, corn syrup, fructose, honey, and turbinado (purified in the same manner as white sugar, but not all of the molasses has been removed).

In choosing a dietitic sweetener for my recipes I use fructose. Fructose is a pure carbohydrate made from natural fruit sugars. It is highly processed and is no more nutritious than sucrose (white sugars); yet it has half the carbohydrates. It is available in health food stores in granulated and liquid form, and is about twice as sweet as refined sugar. It is also more expensive.

The most important advantage of fructose is that it requires no immediate insulin for the body's assimilation process and so is absorbed over a longer period of time, ensuring that most of it is used for energy.

Raw honey also produces somewhat the same insulin reaction as fructose, and is said to be more nutritious. However, the nutrients, in average consumption, are very insignificant when compared to minimum daily requirements. You would have to eat a lot of honey to get any substantial nutrients. That's the drawback to honey since it is higher in calories and carbohydrates than both sucrose and fructose.

I must stress here that I don't claim fructose as a nutritional substitute for refined white sugar. The elimination of all processed sugar is the ideal situation. Yet, those of us who were raised on sugar since birth find it the hardest area to overcome, so in the long-run goal to completely change your eating habits and completely do without any form of sugar, fructose is the most obvious choice in sweeteners. The following comparison establishes this:

Type of Sugar (Sweetener)	Unit of Measure	Calories	Carbohydrates
White refined sugar	1 T.	46	11.9
Honey (Strained)	1 T.	61	16.5
Fructose	1 T.	54	9

BODYBUILDING SUPPLEMENTS

You can ask 10 different bodybuilders what supplements to take and I guarantee you will get 10 different answers. Although frustrating at times to the novice bodybuilder trying to learn the ropes, there is a logical reason for this. As we learned earlier, each metabolism is unique. Thus each program will also be unique. There is no one program that will suit everyone.

It can seem like a complicated puzzle at times, but designing your personal vitamin and mineral program is an important step in perfecting your overall physique.

A very important reminder: in taking supplements, they should be introduced in gradually increasing doses.

A good bodybuilding supplement program, and the one that Pat Neve follows, should include: Vitamin A (with D). All the B vitamins (biotin, inosital, folic acid, paraaminobenzoic acid and choline). Also Vitamin C, Vitamin E, Calcium (with phosphorus), Iron and/or Desiccated Liver, Magnesium, Potassium and Zinc.

Brewer's yeast and desiccated liver are two of the most vital food concentrates employed in Pat Neve's diet.

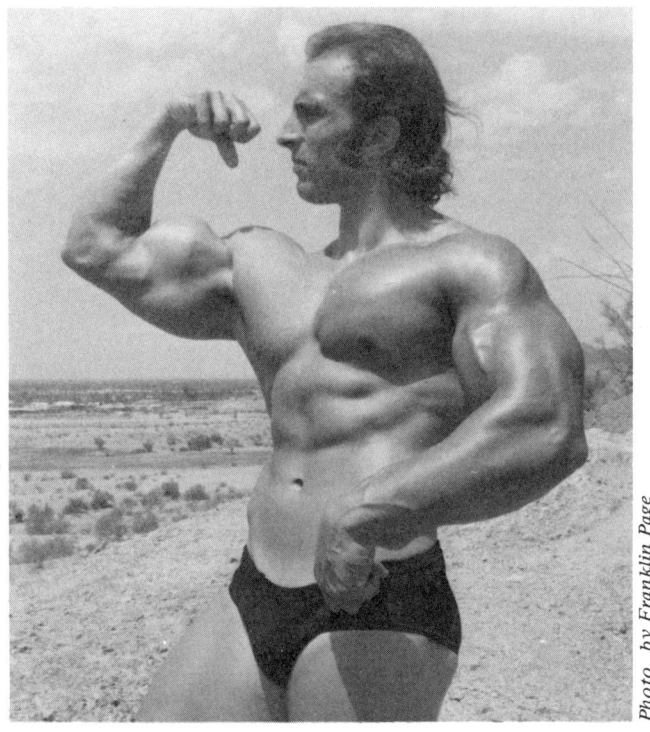

PAT, 24, TRAINING FOR MR. USA

NATURAL VS. SYNTHETIC VITAMINS

There is a continuous debate over the use of synthetic or natural vitamins. Personally, I feel both forms are acceptable. While synthetic vitamins serve the immediate purpose, there are added benefits to taking natural-source vitamins. The natural vitamins often contain both known and unknown nutrients which the synthetic vitamins lack.

I have not read any conclusive evidence against synthetic vitamins being useful, and they are usually smaller and easier to take — and they cost less than natural vitamins.

Pat's personal vitamin program is a combination of both natural and synthetic vitamins, relying specifically on a natural form of Vitamin C with rose hips, and natural Vitamin E (D-alpha tocopherol).

FOOD CONCENTRATES

Because we do not always follow a balanced diet, food concentrates can fill certain nutritional gaps in our diets. There are real, significant improvements in our health when we take daily doses of desiccated liver, lecithin, wheat germ, brewer's yeast and yogurt, etc.

They are most effective in substantial amounts, adding nutrients deficient in your diet, and providing certain foods in a more acceptable form. For example, those who dislike liver often do not object to taking desiccated liver as a diet supplement. Remember that food concentrates have calories, read the label information, and adjust your diet accordingly.

DIURETICS AND THE BODYBUILDER

The final touch in definition is removing all excess body fluid. This can sometimes be accomplished through a combination of Vitamin B6 and Vitamin C. The sun is also a valuable asset in this area. By utilizing the sun for dehydration, the skin becomes thinner and tighter. Also the physique looks harder when tanned, so don't ignore the usefulness of the sun as a vital aid in the overall training program.

VASCULARITY

Here again diet can play a key role in developing those last minute finishing touches. The day of competition a bodybuilder should eat an extra 75 to 100 grams of carbohydrates. Through body processes, these extra carbohydrates cause the blood to rush through the veins, creating the ever popular vascular appearance.

These extra carbohydrates should be in the form of raw fruits, and perhaps two or three tablespoons of fructose. Take the fructose by itself, not added to a drink, to avoid bloating.

PAT, 25, AT JUNIOR USA CONTEST, PLACED 3RD

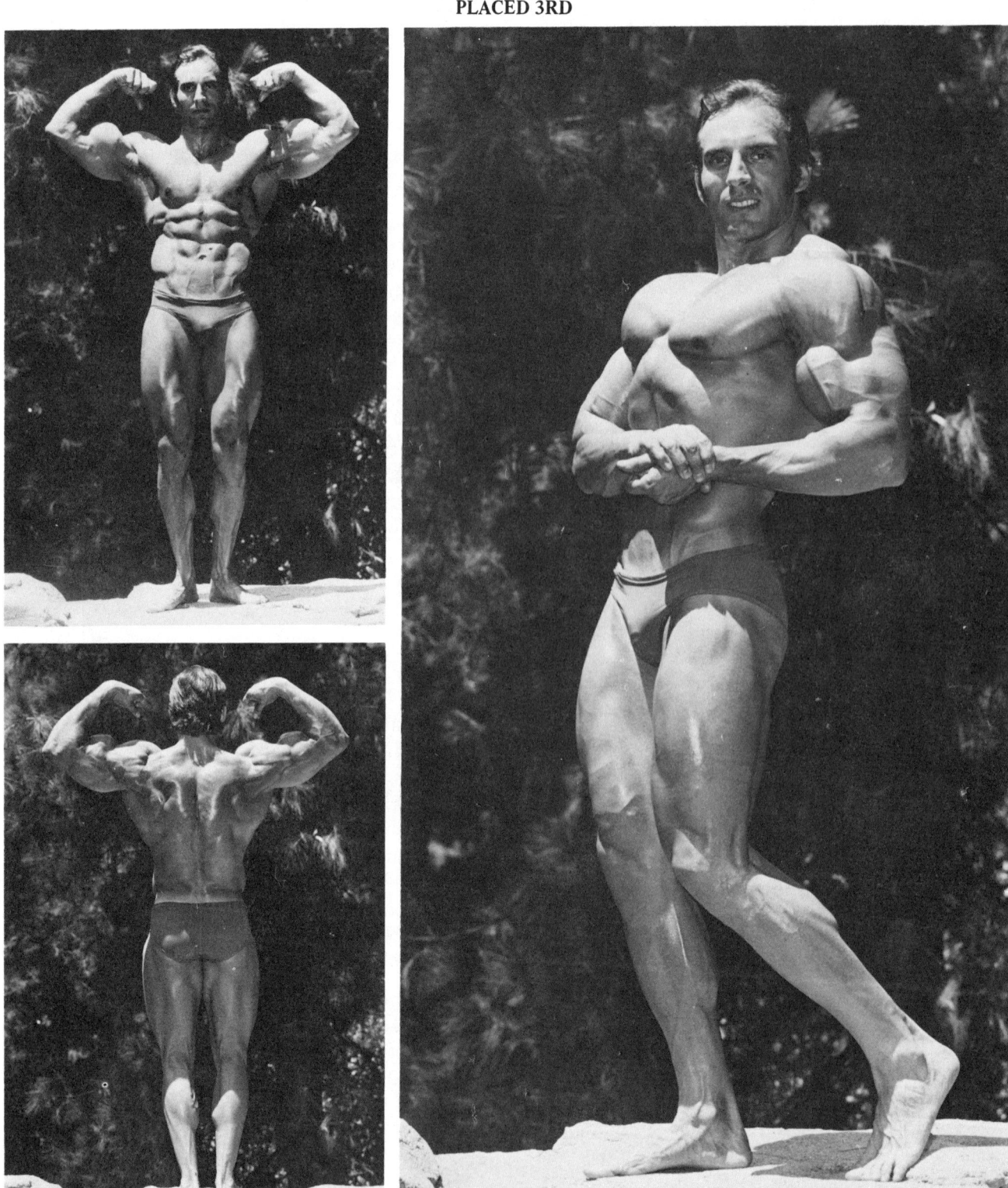

Photos by Dave Sauer

IV
14-DAY WEIGHT-LOSS DIET and MENUS

Basically, this program consists of a low carbohydrate diet that is high in protein and moderate in fats. It is made up of three individual programs to insure total success:
1) The diet program
2) The exercise program
3) The supplement program

The Diet Program limits the daily carbohydrate intake to 50 grams or less. All white refined sugar and flour products are completely eliminated. Most dairy products are limited, with the exception of cheese. The dairy products can be reintroduced in moderation on the **Maintaining Diet** discussed later.

Some might argue that these restrictions are vitamin deficient, yet it is my opinion that an overweight condition is a much more serious health hazard. An obvious solution to any short-range vitamin shortage is through vitamin supplements. These restrictions are necessary in accelerating the weight loss as quickly and comfortably as possible.

A good nationally advertised multiple vitamin is recommended, along with extra Vitamin C, Vitamin E and B-complex. Refer to the vitamin and mineral guide in the back of this book on how to take supplements properly.

Last but by no means least important, is the exercise program. You **will not** see any substantial weight loss without exercise. The whole idea in weight reducing is to burn up more calories as energy than are being consumed in your daily diet. Through exercise you not only burn excess calories, but depending on the type and intensity of the excercise, you can burn off the fat already stored in the body.

I recommend some form of aerobic exercise such as jogging, running in place or jumping rope to produce the fastest overall loss in body fat, especially subcutaneous fat such as cellulite that forms on top of the muscle just under the skin. Of course, in bodybuilding, the weight-resisting exercise is also a must. It isolates each muscle group, building strength, muscle mass and growth. Weight-resisting exercise will also attack the intramuscular fat by working the muscle. But here again a fairly new theory in the benefits to aerobic exercise should not be overlooked as a more thorough way to burn off all body fat, whereas weight-resisting exercise generally only reduces fat in the muscle itself.

The basic diet format includes three meals a day. These meals should consist primarily of poultry or fish, low carbohydrate fruits and vegetables, eggs and cheese. Beef, lamb and veal, etc. may be eaten two-three times a week. Reduce your salt intake as much as possible and do not eat after 7:00 p.m.

Another helpful hint is to eat slowly. This not only aids digestion but will help you feel more satisfied on less food.

PAT,
27,
MR. AMERICA
OF
1975

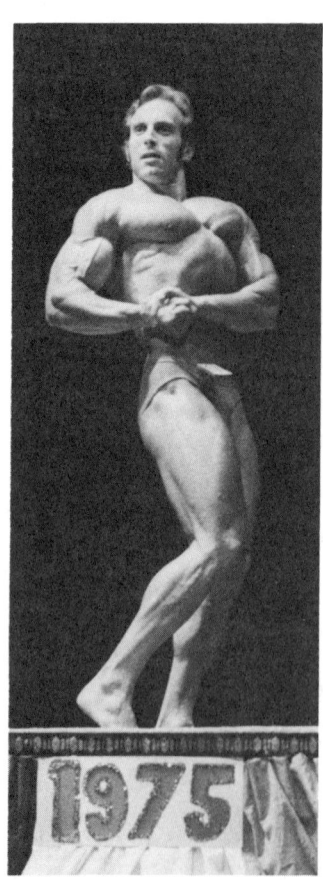
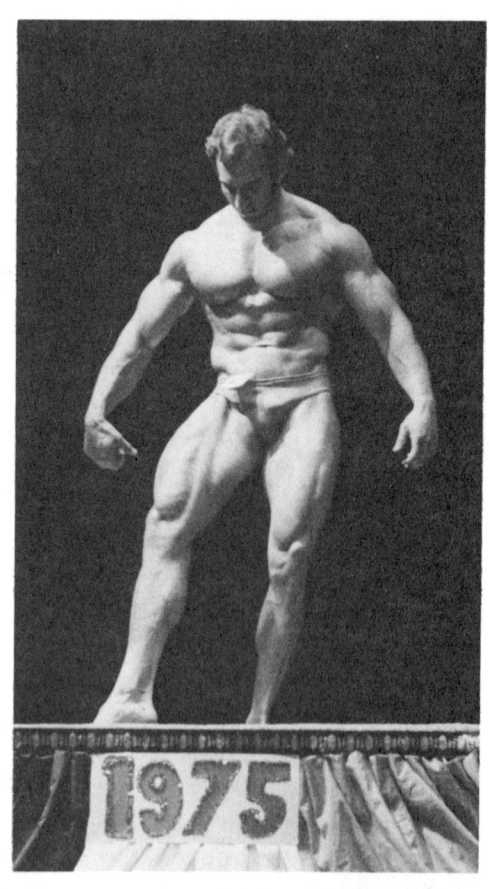
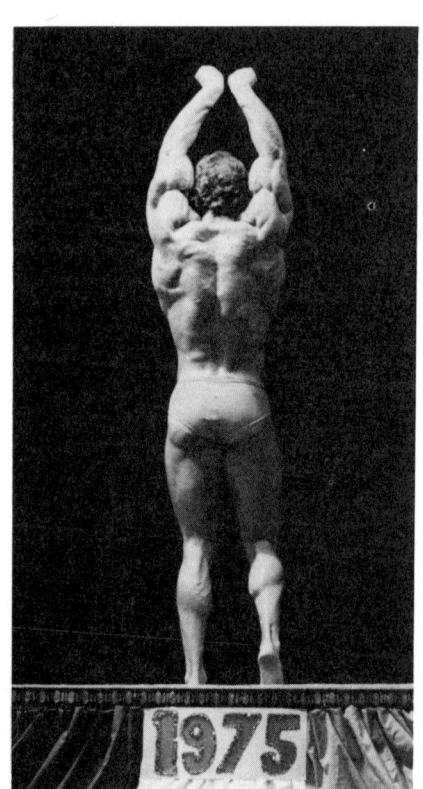
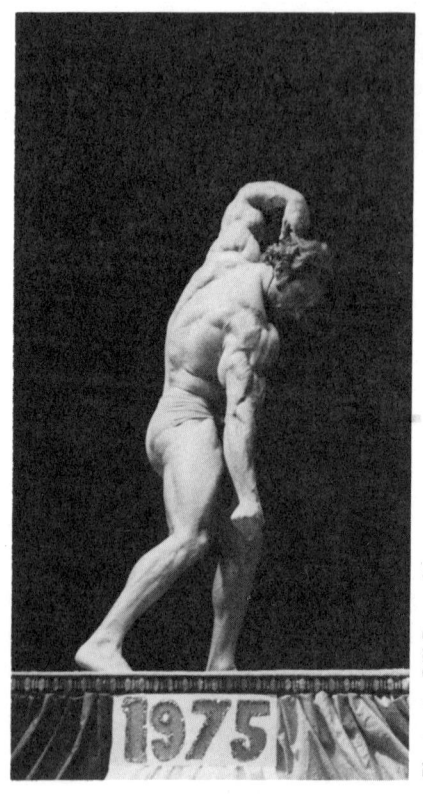
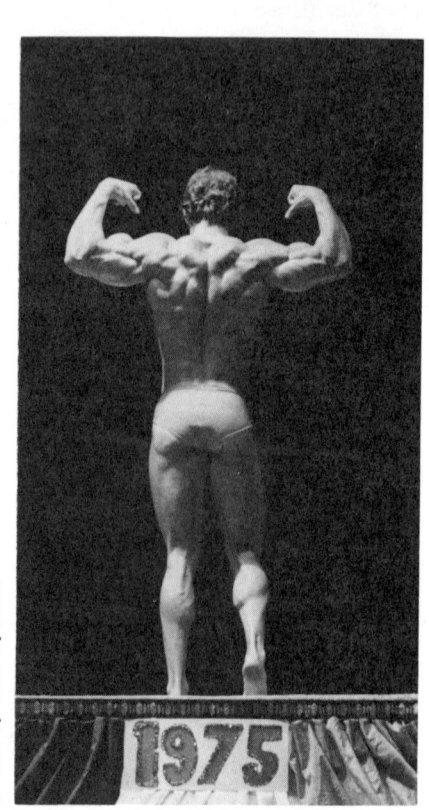

Photos by Bill Reynolds

1st DAY	Approximate Carbohydrates
BREAKFAST	
1-2 eggs, any style	trace
1 cup fresh cantalope	12
Decaffeinated coffee or tea	0
LUNCH	
1 cup Tuna Salad, pg. 53	5
2 Stuffed Eggs, pg. 53	trace
Spiced Tea, pg. 65	0
DINNER	
Cod and Cheese Sauce, pg. 62	trace
Dinner Salad w/choice of dressing pg. 54	5
½ cup Gingered Carrots pg. 55	5
Perrier Water	trace
	27

2nd Day	Approximate Carbohydrates
BREAKFAST	
1-2 eggs, any style	trace
1 cup fresh strawberries	12
w/1 tsp. fructose (optional)	(5)
Decaffeinated coffee or tea	0
LUNCH	
1 cup Hearty Beef Salad, pg. 53	5
2 oz. cheese	1
Iced coffee, pg. 65	0
DINNER	
Tarragon Chicken in Wine	1
Dinner Salad w/choice of dressing, pg. 54	5
Cheese Tomato Broil, pg. 56	6
Spiced Tea, pg. 65	0
	35

3rd Day	Approximate Carbohydrates
BREAKFAST	
1-2 eggs, any style	trace
1 med. fresh peach or ¾ cup frozen peaches, unsw.	12
Decaffeinated coffee or tea	0
LUNCH	
1 Cup Turkey Salad, pg. 53	5
Iced Tea	0
DINNER	
Tropical Chicken, pg. 61	trace
Dinner Salad w/choice of dressing, pg. 54	5
3/4 cup Seasoned Green Beans, pg. 56	5
Perrier Water	0
	27

4th Day	Approximate Carbohydrates
BREAKFAST	
1-2 eggs, any style	trace
1 cup diced honeydew melon	12.9
Decaffeinated coffee or tea	0
LUNCH	
1 cup Shrimp Salad, pg. 53	5
2 pc. Stuffed Celery, pg. 52	3
Iced Coffee, pg. 65	0
DINNER	
Stuffed Game Hen, pg. 61	5
Dinner Salad, w/choice of dressing, pg. 54	5
1 cup Cauliflower w/cheese pg. 56	5
Perrier Water	0
	35.9

5th Day

	Approximate Carbohydrates
BREAKFAST	
1-2 eggs, any style	trace
1 cup fresh strawberries	12
or unsweetened frozen	
w/1 tsp. fructose (optional)	(5)
LUNCH	
1 Cheeseburger, pg. 57	5
2 Stuffed Eggs, pg. 53	trace
Iced Tea	0
DINNER	
1 serving Turkey Oscar, pg. 60	2
3/4 cup Spinach &	
Broccoli, pg. 56	5
Dinner Salad w/choice of	
dressing, pg. 54	5
Spiced Tea, pg. 65	0
	29

6th Day

	Approximate Carbohydrates
BREAKFAST	
1-2 eggs, any style	trace
1 medium fresh peach or	
unsweetened frozen peaches	12
Decaffeinated coffee or tea	0
LUNCH	
1 cup Fresh Mushroom	
Salad, pg. 53	5
2 Stuffed Eggs, pg. 52	trace
Iced Coffee, pg. 65	0
DINNER	
1 serving Parmesan	
Chicken, pg. 61	trace
3 Stuffed Mushrooms, pg. 53	4
Dinner Salald w/choice of	
dressing, pg.54	5
Spiced Tea, pg. 65	0
	26

7th Day

	Approximate Carbohydrates
BREAKFAST	
1-2 eggs, any style	trace
1 cup fresh cantaloupe	12
(or frozen, if available)	
Decaffeinated coffee or tea	0
LUNCH	
1 cup Hot Spinach	
Salad, pg. 52	5
(3) Egg Toppers, pg. 51	3
Iced Tea	0
DINNER	
1 serving Prime Rib, pg. 58	0
1 cup Skillet Zucchini, pg. 55	3
Dinner Salad w/choice of	
dressing, pg. 54	5
Perrier Water	0
	28

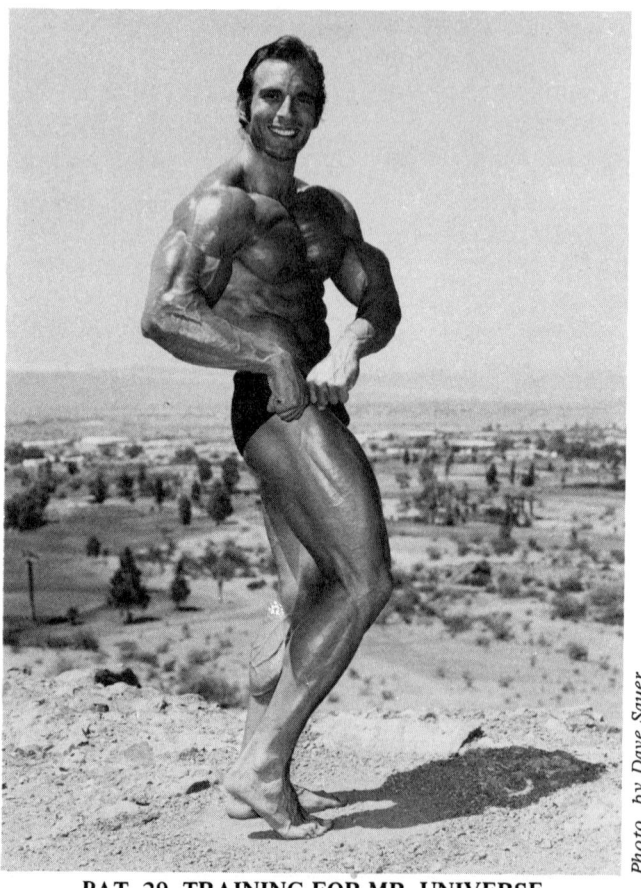

PAT, 29, TRAINING FOR MR. UNIVERSE

Photo by Dave Sauer

8th Day — Approximate Carbohydrates

BREAKFAST
- 1-2 eggs, any style — trace
- 1 cup fresh honeydew melon (or frozen, if not available) — 12.9
- Decaffeinated coffee or tea — 0

LUNCH
- Stuffed Tomato, pg. 56 — 7
- Iced Coffee, pg. 65 — 0

DINNER
- 1 serving Chicken & Mushrooms, pg. 61 — trace
- Dinner Salad w/choice of dressing, pg. 54 — 5
- 1 cup Broiled Zucchini Chips, pg. 51 — 3
- Perrier Water, pg. 65 — 0

Total: 27.9

9th Day — Approximate Carbohydrates

BREAKFAST
- 1-2 eggs, any style — trace
- 1 medium fresh peach or unsweetened frozen — 12
- Decaffeinated coffee or tea — 0

LUNCH
- 1 cup Fruit Salad, pg. 53 — 7
- Iced Tea — 0

DINNER
- 1 cup Onion Soup, pg. 52 — 5
- 1 Broiled Lobster Tail, pg. 62 — trace
- Dinner Salad w/choice of dressing, pg. 54 — 5
- Spiced Tea — 0

Total: 29

10th Day — Approximate Carbohydrates

BREAKFAST
- 1-2 eggs any style — trace
- 1 cup fresh Cantaloupe (or frozen, if available) — 12
- Decaffeinated coffee or tea — 0

LUNCH
- (1) 3 inch wedge Quiche, pg. 54 — 5
- Guacamole Stuffed Celery, pg. 52 — 3
- Iced Tea — 0

DINNER
- 1 serving Marinated London Broil, pg. 60 — 4
- (3) Stuffed Mushrooms, pg. 56 — 4
- Dinner Salad, w/choice of dressing, pg. 54 — 5
- Perrier Water — 0

Total: 29

11th Day — Approximate Carbohydrates

BREAKFAST
- 1-2 eggs, any style — trace
- 1 cup fresh strawberries or unsweetened frozen — 12
- Decaffeinated coffee or tea — 0

LUNCH
- 1 cup raw Vegetable Soup, pg. 52 — 5
- 2 Stuffed Eggs, pg. 52 — Trace
- Spiced Tea, pg. 65 — 0

DINNER
- 1 serving Baked Fish, Piquant, pg. 62 — trace
- Dinner Salad w/choice of dressing, pg. 54 — 5
- Marinated Cucumbers & Onions, pg. 55 — 5
- Perrier Water — 0

Total: 27

12th Day	Approximate Carbohydrates
BREAKFAST	
1-2 eggs, any style	trace
1 medium fresh peach or unsweetened frozen	12
Decaffeinated coffee or tea	0
LUNCH	
1 cup Bacon and Egg Salad pg. 53	5
2 pc. Guacamole Stuffed Celery, pg. 52	3
Iced Tea	0
DINNER	
1 serving Veal & Sour Cream pg. 60	trace
1 cup Spinach, pg. 56	5
Dinner Salad w/choice of dressing, pg. 54	5
Iced Coffee, pg. 65	0
	30

13th Day	Approximate Carbohydrates
BREAKFAST	
1-2 eggs, any style	trace
1 cup fresh honeydew melon (or frozen, if available)	12.9
Decaffeinated coffee or tea	0
LUNCH	
1 cup Peach and Cheese Salad, pg. 53	10
Iced Tea	0
DINNER	
1 serving Shrimp Delight pg. 62	trace
Dinner Salad w/choice of dressing, pg. 54	5
1 cup Cauliflower w/cheese, pg. 56	5
Perrier Water	0
	22.9

14th Day	Approximate Carbohydrates
BREAKFAST	
1-2 eggs, any style	trace
1 cup fresh cantaloupe or frozen, if available	12
Decaffeinated coffee or tea	0
LUNCH	
Mexiburger, pg. 58	5
Iced Tea	0
DINNER	
1 serving Salmon Steaks pg. 62	0
1 cup Seasoned Green Beans, pg. 56	5
Dinner Salad w/choice of dressing, pg. 54	5
Spiced Tea, pg. 65	0
	27

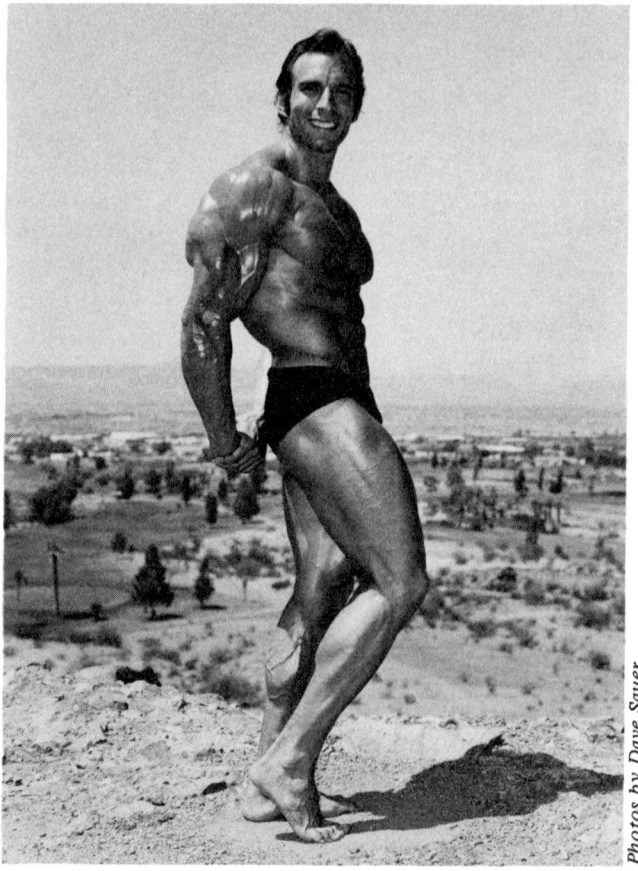

PAT, 29, TRAINING FOR MR. UNIVERSE

Photos by Dave Sauer

V
14-DAY WEIGHT-GAIN DIET and MENUS

*T*he object of most novice bodybuilders is to gain muscular size. The mistake many make is in the assumption that gaining weight is simply a matter of increasing their calorie intake, primarily on high calorie junk foods. Many of our gym members confess to this practice, and gave us the sample daily menu which follows as a typical example of their weight gain attempts.

BREAKFAST	LUNCH	DINNER
Pancakes (unlimited quantities)	2 Super-burgers (from various fast-food establishments)	Spaghetti and Meatballs
Sausage		Garlic Toast
Hash brown potatoes	2 orders French Fried Potatoes	Salad
Milk (2 or 3 glasses)	Chocolate Milkshake	Cola (2 or 3 glasses)
		Cake for dessert

On this type of diet you will gain weight all right, most of it in your stomach! This diet simply creates body fat, NOT muscular weight. To gain solid muscular weight takes a precise diet just as important as a weight-loss diet. Don't give up quality for quantity.

Most experts agree that approximately 5 to 7 pounds of pure muscle can be gained in one year. So, the young athlete who gains 20 pounds in 2 months on junk foods can be assured that a large percentage of extra body weight is fat, not muscle. You don't create muscle on junk foods. Muscle growth and development comes only with a dedicated, consistent application of weight training, diet and supplement program. The weight-gain diet and supplement program in this book sets the nutritional standards and atmosphere to accommodate the vigorous weight-training needed for muscle development.

Pat put each of our members who wanted to gain weight on the following diet plan, along with the weight-gain supplement program, with amazing results. Each and every member gained 2 to 4 pounds a week, THE RIGHT WAY.

PAT NEVE'S WEIGHT GAIN SUPPLEMENT PROGRAM

- 15   Dessicated liver tablets - 10½ grains (3-5 times a day)
- 15   Brewer's Yeast tablets - 12 grains (3-5 times a day)
- 2   Milk and Egg protein drinks (Mix 2 tablespoons powered milk and egg protein with whole milk, to take before and after the workout.

1st DAY

BREAKFAST
- 3-4 Eggs, any style
- 4 oz. Canadian Bacon
- 1 pc. Whole Wheat Toast with Honey
- 4 oz. Fruit Juice
- Weight-gain protein drink, pg. 27

MID-MORNING
- Peanut Butter Sandwich with Banana or Honey
- 8 oz. Whole Milk

LUNCH
- Stuffed Burger, pg. 57
- ½ cup Cottage Cheese
- 8 oz. Whole Milk

MID-AFTERNOON
- 8 oz. Yogurt, any flavor
- Weight-gain protein drink, pg. 27

DINNER
- Veal and Sour Cream, pg. 60
- Skillet Zucchini, pg. 55
- Salad
- 1 pc. Whole Wheat Bread with Butter
- 8 oz. Whole Milk

EARLY EVENING
- Jello and Fruit
- 8 oz. Whole Milk

2nd DAY

BREAKFAST
- 3-4 Eggs, any style
- 1 pc. Whole Wheat Toast with Butter
- 3 pcs. Sausage
- 4 oz. Fruit Juice
- Weight-gain protein drink, pg. 27

MID-MORNING
- 8 oz. Yogurt, any flavor
- 8 oz. Whole Milk

LUNCH
- Tuna Salad, pg. 53
- ½ cup Cottage Cheese
- 8 oz. Whole Milk

MID-AFTERNOON
- Cheese and Fresh Raw Vegetables
- Weight-gain protein drink, pg. 27

DINNER
- Zippy Lamb Shanks, pg. 63
- Salad
- Zucchini Chips, pg. 51
- Weight-gain protein drink, pg. 27

EARLY EVENING
- Fruit and Jello
- 8 oz. Whole Milk

3rd DAY

BREAKFAST
- Breakfast Steak
- 3 Eggs, any style
- 4 oz. Fruit Juice
- Weight-gain protein drink, pg.00

MID-MORNING
- 1 cup Cottage Cheese
- 1 pc. of Fruit
- 8 oz. Whole Milk

LUNCH
- Ham Salad
- 8 oz. Whole Milk

MID- AFTERNOON
- Dried Fruits, Apricots, Apples, Raisins, etc.
- Nuts
- Weight-gain protein drink, pg. 27

DINNER
- Ribbon Meat Loaf, pg. 59
- Baked Potato with Butter and Sour Cream
- Cheese Broiled Asparagus, pg. 56
- 8 oz. Whole Milk

EARLY EVENING
- 1 pc. Toast with Peanut Butter and Honey
- 8 oz. Whole Milk

4th DAY

BREAKFAST
   3-4 Eggs, any style
   3 pc. Sausage
   1 pc. Whole Wheat Toast with Honey
   4 oz. Fruit Juice
   Weight-gain protein drink, pg. 27

MID-MORNING
   Stuffed Burger, pg. 57
   8 oz. Whole Milk

LUNCH
   Broiled Steak
   2 Scrambled Eggs
   ½ cup Cottage Cheese
   8 oz. Whole Milk

MID-AFTERNOON
   Fruits and Nuts
   Weight-gain protein drink, pg. 27

DINNER
   Ribbon Meat Loaf, pg. 59
   Baked Potato with Sour Cream and Butter
   Corn
   Salad
   8 oz. Whole Milk

EARLY EVENING
   Jello
   8 oz. Whole Milk

5th DAY

BREAKFAST
   Oatmeal with Whole Milk and Fructose
   1 pc. Whole Wheat Toast
   2 pcs. Bacon
   4 oz. Fruit Juice
   Weight-gain protein drink, pg. 27

MID-MORNING
   Hearty Beef Salad, pg. 53
   ½ cup Cottage Cheese
   8oz. Whole Milk

LUNCH
   Stuffed Burger, pg. 57
   8 oz. Whole Milk

MID-AFTERNOON
   Peanut Butter and Honey Sandwich
      on Whole Wheat
   Weight-gain protein drink, pg. 27

DINNER
   Roast Beef with Gravy
   Salad
   1 cup Carrots
   8 oz. Whole Milk

EARLY EVENING
   8 oz. Yogurt
   8 oz. Whole Milk

6th DAY

BREAKFAST
   3-4 Eggs, any style
   3 pcs. Sausage
   1 pc. Whole Wheat Toast with Butter
   4 oz. Fruit Juice
   Weight-gain protein drink, pg. 27

MID-MORNING
   8 oz. Yogurt, any flavor
   8 oz. Whole Milk

MID-AFTERNOON
   1 Banana
   ½ cup Cottage Cheese
   Weight-gain protein drink, pg. 27

DINNER
   Prime Rib, pg. 58
   Baked Potato with Butter and Sour Cream
   Salad
   Broccoli
   8 oz. Whole Milk

EARLY EVENING
   Dried Fruits and Nuts
   8 oz. Whole Milk

7th DAY

BREAKFAST
- 3-4 Eggs, any style
- ¼ lb. Ground Beef Patty
- 1 pc. Whole Wheat Toast with Butter
- 4 oz. Fruit Juice
- Weight-gain protein drink, pg. 27

MID-MORNING
- Peanut Butter Sandwich with Honey on Whole Wheat
- 8 oz. Whole Milk

LUNCH
- Turkey Salad, pg. 53
- ½ cup Cottage Cheese
- 8 oz. Whole Milk

MID-AFTERNOON
- 8 oz. Yogurt, any flavor
- Weight-gain protein drink, pg. 27

DINNER
- Baked Fish, pg. 62
- 1 cup Seasoned Green Beans, pg. 56
- 1 Baked Potato with Butter and Sour Cream
- 8 oz. Whole Milk

EARLY EVENING
- 4 oz. Cheese, any kind
- Nuts
- 1 pc. Fruit
- 8 oz. Whole Milk

8th Day

BREAKFAST
- Cold Cereal with Whole Milk and Fructose (preferably Granola type)
- 2 pc. Bacon
- 4 oz. Fruit Juice
- Weight-gain protein drink

MID-MORNING
- 8 oz. Yogurt, any flavor
- 8 oz. Whole Milk

LUNCH
- ½ lb. Ground Beef Patty with Melted Cheese
- Salad
- 8 oz. Whole Milk

MID-AFTERNOON
- 1 Banana
- ½ cup Cottage Cheese
- Weight-gain protein drink, pg. 27

DINNER
- Steak
- ¾ cup Brussel Sprouts
- Salad
- 8 oz. Whole Milk

EARLY EVENING
- Jello and Fruit
- 8 oz. Whole Milk

9th DAY

BREAKFAST
- Cooked Cream of Wheat Cereal with Whole Milk
- 1 pc. Whole Wheat Toast with Butter
- 4 oz. Fruit Juice
- Weight-gain protein drink, pg. 27

MID-MORNING
- Stuffed Burger, pg. 57
- 8 oz. Whole Milk

LUNCH
- Cube Steak
- ½ cup Cottage Cheese
- 8 oz. Whole Milk

MID-AFTERNOON
- 8 oz. Yogurt, any flavor
- Weight-gain protein drink, pg. 27

DINNER
- Parmesan Chicken, pg. 61
- 1 cup Cauliflower, with Cheese Sauce, pg. 56
- Salad
- 8 oz. Whole Milk

EARLY EVENING
    1 pc. Fruit and Cheese
    8 oz. Whole Milk

10th DAY

BREAKFAST
    3-4 Eggs, any style
    1 pc. Whole Wheat Toast with Butter
    2 pcs. Bacon
    4 oz. Fruit Juice
    Weight-gain protein drink, pg. 27

MID-MORNING
    Cold Chicken or Turkey
    8 oz. Whole Milk

LUNCH
    Shrimp Salad, pg. 53
    ½ cup Cottage Cheese
    8 oz. Whole Milk

MID-AFTERNOON
    8 oz. Yogurt, any flavor
    Weight-gain protein drink, pg. 27

DINNER
    Lemon Pot Roast, pg. 59
    Stuffed Mushrooms, pg. 56
    Salad
    Baked Egg Custard, pg. 65
    8 oz. Whole Milk

EARLY EVENING
    1 pc. Whole Wheat Toast with Peanut Butter
    8 oz. Whole Milk

11th DAY

BREAKFAST
    Cold Cereal with Whole Milk and Fructose
      (preferably Granola type)
    3 pcs. Bacon
    1 pc. Whole Wheat Toast with Butter
    4 oz. Fruit Juice
    Weight-gain protein drink, pg. 27

MID-MORNING
    Cold Roast Beef or Chicken
    8 oz. Whole Milk

LUNCH
    Bacon and Egg Salad, pg. 53
    8 oz. Whole Milk

MID-AFTERNOON
    Baked Apple with Ricotta, pg. 65
    Weight-gain protein drink, pg. 27

DINNER
    Veal and Sour Cream, pg. 60
    Stuffed Tomatoes, pg. 56
    Salad
    8 oz. Whole Milk

EARLY EVENING
    ½ cup Cottage Cheese
    1 pc. Fruit
    8 oz. Whole Milk

12th DAY

BREAKFAST
    3-4 Eggs, any style
    Breakfast Steak
    1 pc. Whole Wheat Toast with Butter
    4 oz. Fruit Juice
    Weight-gain protein drink, pg. 27

MID-MORNING
    8 oz. Yogurt, any flavor
    8 oz. Whole Milk

LUNCH
    Turkey Oscar, pg. 60
    8 oz. Whole Milk

MID-AFTERNOON
    Jello and Fruit
    Weight-gain protein drink, pg. 27

DINNER
    Lamb Steaks in Marinade, pg. 63
    Salad

Gingered Carrots
8 oz. Whole Milk

EARLY EVENING
Baked Apple Ricotta, pg. 65
8 oz. Whole Milk

13th DAY

BREAKFAST
3-4 Eggs, any style
2 pcs. Bacon
1 pc. Whole Wheat Toast with Butter
4 oz. Fruit Juice
Weight-gain protein drink, pg. 27

MID-MORNING
½ Cantaloupe with Cottage Cheese
8 oz. Whole Milk

LUNCH
Tuna Salad, pg. 53
2 Stuffed Eggs, pg. 52
8 oz. Whole Milk

MID-AFTERNOON
8 oz. Yogurt, any flavor
Weight-gain protein drink

DINNER
Stuffed Peppers, pg. 57
Seasoned Green Beans, pg. 56
Salad
8 oz. Whole Milk

EARLY EVENING
Cheese Omelet
8 oz. Whole Milk

14th DAY

BREAKFAST
Cold Cereal with Whole Milk and Fructose
   (preferably Granola type)
3 pcs. Sausage
1 pc. Whole Wheat Toast with Butter
4 oz. Fruit Juice
Weight-gain protein drink, pg. 27

MID-MORNING
1 pc. Whole Wheat Toast with Peanut Butter
8 oz. Whole Milk

LUNCH
Stuffed Burger, pg. 57
8 oz. Whole Milk

MID-AFTERNOON
Jello and Fruit
Weight-gain protein drink, pg. 27

DINNER
Marinated London Broil, pg. 60
Baked Potato with Sour Cream and Butter
Cheese Tomato Broil, pg. 56
Salad
8 oz. Whole Milk

EARLY EVENING
2 oz. Cheese
1 pc. Fruit
8 oz. Whole Milk

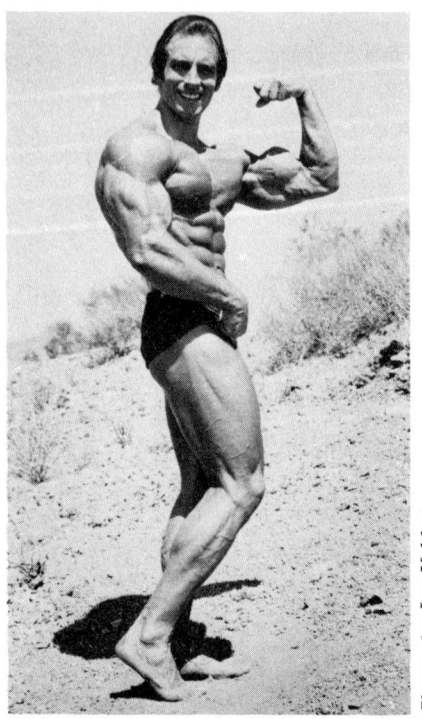

Photo by Joe Valdez

PAT, 30, TRAINING FOR MR. WORLD

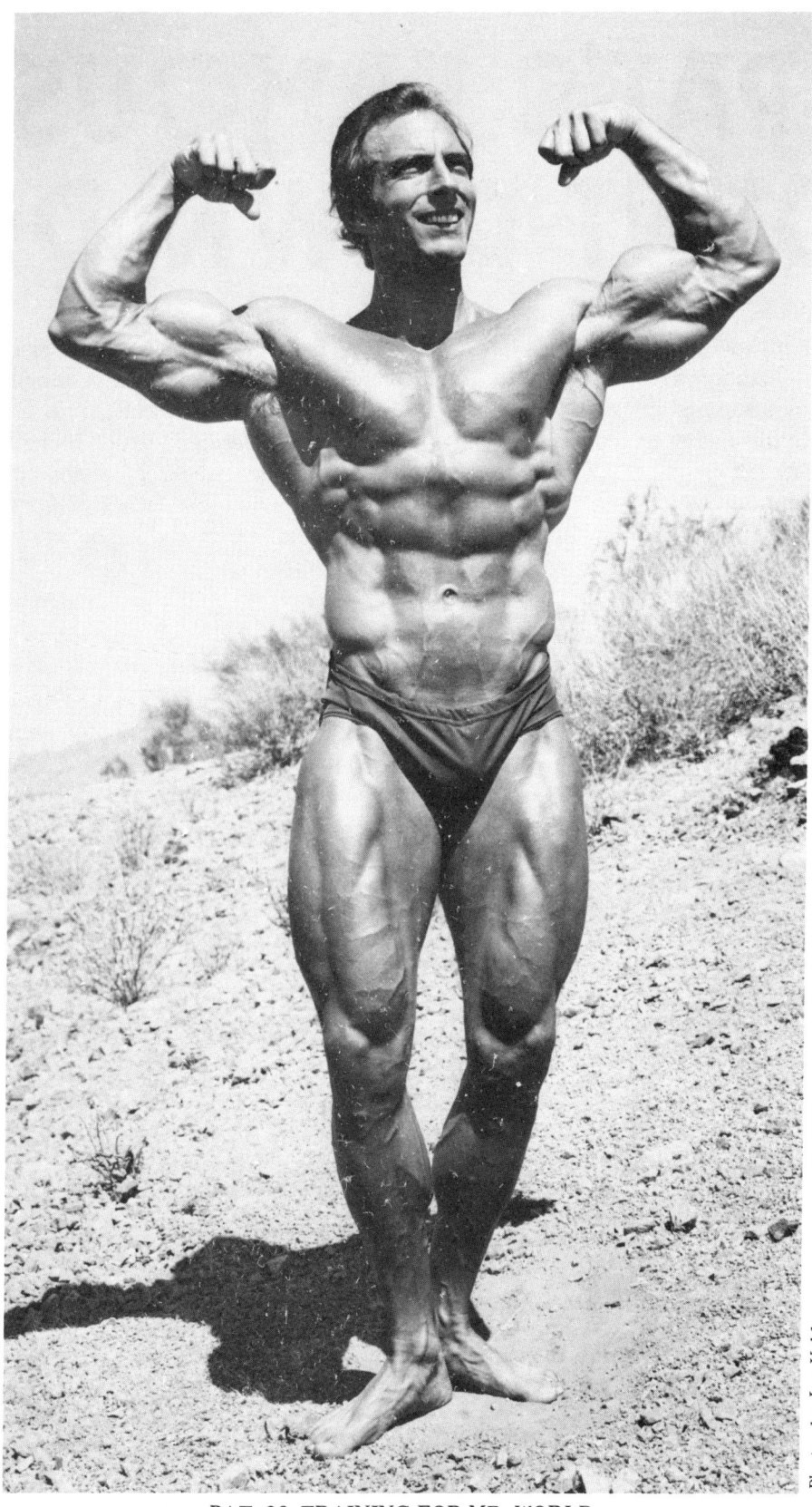

PAT, 30, TRAINING FOR MR. WORLD

Photo by Joe Valdez

VI
PAT'S FAMOUS COUNT-DOWN DIET

On Pat's *Countdown Diet* the idea is to gradually reduce the carbohydrate intake until ultimately you are consuming only enough carbohydrates to supply the energy to train without adding any excess body fat.

You will want to eat five or six smaller meals spaced evenly throughout the day to properly utilize the energy and protein content. During the first three weeks of the five-week countdown period these meals consist of eggs, meat, fowl, fish, cheese and low carbohydrate fruit and vegetables. In an accelerated effort to reduce total calories, the last two weeks of meals consist only of eggs, fowl, fish and low carbohydrate vegetables.

Summarized, the *Countdown Diet* consists of the following:

THE COUNTDOWN DIET

Weeks Prior to Competition	Meal Make-up	Daily Carbohydrate Intake
5 Weeks	Eggs Meat (Beef, Lamb, and Liver) Fowl (Chicken and Turkey) Fish Cheese Fruits and Vegetables (Low Carbohydrate)	50 Grams
4 Weeks	Eggs Meat (Beef, Lamb and Liver) Fowl (Chicken and Turkey) Fish and Cheese Fruits and Vegetables (Low Carbohydrate)	40 Grams
3 Weeks	Eggs Meat (Beef, Lamb and Liver) Fowl (Chicken and Turkey) Fish and Cheese Fruits and Vegetables (Low Carbohydrate)	30 Grams
2 Weeks	Eggs Fowl (Chicken and Turkey) Fish and Cheese Vegetables (Low Carbohydrate)	20 Grams

THE COUNTDOWN DIET (continued)

Weeks Prior to Competition	Meal Make-up	Daily Carbohydrate Intake
1 Week	Eggs Fowl (Chicken and Turkey) Fish and Cheese Vegetables (Low Carbohydrate)	10 Grams

THE DAILY MENUS

5th WEEK

FIRST DAY

BREAKFAST — Carbohydrates

3 eggs, any style or cholesterol free egg substitutes (usually equal in protein, lower in calories and fat and slightly higher in carbohydrates than whole eggs).	1.2
¼ pound ground beef patty	.0
1 cup fresh strawberries	12.0

MID-MORNING

Tuna salad, pg. 53	5.0
2 stuffed eggs, pg. 52	trace

LUNCH

Cornish hen, pg. 61	6.0
½ cup fresh cantaloupe	6.0

MID-AFTERNOON

Omelet, pg. 55	2.0

DINNER

Prime Rib, pg. 58	.0
Dinner salad	5.0
Stuffed mushrooms, pg. 56	5.0

EARLY EVENING

3 eggs, any style	1.2
½ cup fresh cantaloupe	6.0

Total Daily Carbohydrates 49.4

SECOND DAY

BREAKFAST — Carbohydrates

3 eggs, any style	1.2
Sliced roast beef	.0
1 fresh peach	12.0

MID-MORNING

Turkey salad, pg. 53	5.0

LUNCH

Stuffed burger, pg. 57	trace
Lite salad, pg. 53	3.0
1 cup fresh strawberries	12.0

MID-AFTERNOON

Omelet, pg. 55	2.0

DINNER

London broil, pg. 60	trace
Seasoned green beans, pg. 56	4.0
Dinner salad	5.0

EARLY EVENING

3 eggs, any style	1.2
½ cup fresh cantaloupe	6.0

Total Carbohydrates 50.4

THIRD DAY   Carbohydrates

BREAKFAST

3 Eggs, any style	1.2
Breakfast steak	.0
1 cup fresh strawberries	12.0

MID-MORNING

Turkey salad, pg. 53	5.0

LUNCH

Parmesan chicken, pg. 61	trace
Dinner salad	5.0
½ cup fresh cantaloupe	6.0

MID-AFTERNOON

Omelet, pg. 55	2.0

DINNER

Roast beef, pg. 58	.0
1 cup asparagus, pg. 56	6.0
Dinner salad	5.0

EARLY EVENING

3 eggs, any style	1.2
½ cup fresh cantaloupe	6.0

Total Daily Carbohydrates 49.4

FOURTH DAY

BREAKFAST

3 eggs, any style	1.2
Cube steak	.0
½ cup fresh cantaloupe	6.0

MID-MORNING

Hearty beef salad, pg. 53	5.0

LUNCH

Liver, pg. 60	1.0
2 stuffed eggs, pg. 52	trace
1 cup fresh strawberries	12.0

MID-AFTERNOON

Omelet, pg. 55	2.0

DINNER

Tarragon chicken, pg. 61	trace
Dinner salad	5.0
Broiled tomatoes, pg. 56	5.0

EARLY EVENING

3 eggs, any style	1.2
1 fresh peach	12.0

Total Daily Carbohydrates 50.4

FIFTH DAY   Carbohydrates

BREAKFAST

3 eggs, any style	1.2
Baked chicken breast	.0
1 cup strawberries	12.0

MID-MORNING

Turkey salad, pg. 53	5.0

LUNCH

Boiled shrimp with lemon butter pg. 62	trace
1 cup cauliflower, pg. 56	5.0
½ cup fresh cantaloupe	6.0

MID AFTERNOON

Omelet, pg. 55	2.0

DINNER

Grilled rib-eye steak	.0
Dinner salad	5.0
½ cup sauteed mushrooms	5.0

EARLY EVENING

3 eggs, any style	1.2
½ cup fresh cantaloupe	6.0

Total Daily Carbohydrates 49.4

NOTE: On Saturday and Sunday, repeat the weekday menu of your choice.

4th WEEK

FIRST DAY

BREAKFAST

3 eggs, any style	1.2
Sliced cold turkey	.0
½ cup fresh strawberries	12.0

MID-MORNING

Tuna salad, pg. 53	5.0

LUNCH

Basic lamb chops, pg. 63	.0
Sliced cucumbers	1.0

MID-AFTERNOON

Omelet, pg. 55	2.0

DINNER

Ribbon meatloaf, pg. 59	trace
1 cup caulifower, pg. 56	5.0

EARLY EVENING

	Carbohydrates
3 eggs, any style	1.2

Total Daily Carbohydrates 38.4

SECOND DAY

BREAKFAST

3 eggs, any style	1.2
Slice roast beef	.0
1 cup of fresh strawberries	12.0

MID-MORNING

Tuna salad, pg. 53	5.0

LUNCH

Stuffed burger, pg. 57	trace
2 stuffed eggs, pg. 52	trace

MID-AFTERNOON

Omelet, pg. 55	2.0
1 fresh peach	12.0

DINNER

Tropical chicken, pg. 61	trace
Lite salad, pg. 53	3.0
1 cup skillet zucchini, pg. 55	4.0

EARLY EVENING

3 eggs, any style	1.2

Total Daily Carbohydrates 40.4

THIRD DAY

BREAKFAST

3 eggs, any style	1.2
Stuffed burger, pg. 57	trace
½ cup fresh cantaloupe	6.0

MID-MORNING

Hot spinach salad, pg. 52	5.0
2 hard-boiled eggs	trace

LUNCH

Liver and onions, pg. 60	1.0
2 slices fresh tomatoes	3.0

MID-AFTERNOON

Omelet, pg. 55	2.0
1 fresh peach	12.0

DINNER

Parmesan chicken, pg. 61	trace
½ cup broccoli & bacon, pg. 55	4.0
Dinner salad	5.0

EARLY EVENING

	Carbohydrates
3 eggs, any style	1.2

Total Daily Carbohydrates 40.4

FOURTH DAY

BREAKFAST

3 eggs, any style	1.2
Breakfast steak	.0
1 fresh peach	12.0

MID-MORNING

Hearty beef salad, pg. 53	5.0
1 raw carrot	4.0

LUNCH

Boiled shrimp with lemon butter, pg. 62	trace
2 stuffed eggs	trace

MID-AFTERNOON

Omelet, pg. 55	2.0
½ cup fresh cantaloupe	6.0

DINNER

Herbed lamb shanks, pg. 63	.0
1 cup seasoned green beans, pg. 56	5.0
Dinner salad	5.0

EARLY EVENING

3 eggs, any style	1.2

Total Daily Carbohydrates 40.4

FIFTH DAY

BREAKFAST

3 eggs, any syle	1.2
1 baked chicken breast	.0
1 cup cantaloupe	12.0

MID MORNING

Turkey salad	5.0
Sliced cucumbers	1.0

LUNCH

Candy's Beef patties	trace
½ cup strawberries	6.0

DINNER

Veal and sour cream	trace
Dinner salad	5.0
1 cup seasoned green beans	6.0

EARLY EVENING	Carbohydrates
3 eggs, any style	1.2

Total Carbohydrates 37.4

NOTE: On Saturday and Sunday, repeat the weekday menu of your choice.

3rd WEEK

FIRST DAY

BREAKFAST

3 eggs, any style	1.2
¼ pound ground beef patty	.0
½ cup fresh cantaloupe	6.0

MID-MORNING

Bacon and egg salad, pg. 53	5.0

LUNCH

Zippy lamb shanks, pg. 63	.0
2 stuffed eggs, pg. 52	trace

MID-AFTERNOON

Omelet, pg. 55	2.0
½ cup fresh cantaloupe	6.0

DINNER

Prime rib, pg. 58	.0
½ cup brussel sprouts	5.0
Dinner salad	5.0

EARLY EVENING

3 eggs, any style	1.2

Total Daily Carbohydrates 31.4

SECOND DAY

BREAKFAST

3 eggs, any style	1.2
¼ pound ground beef patty with melted cheese	trace
1 cup fresh strawberries	12.0

MID-MORNING

Tuna salad, pg. 53	5.0

LUNCH

Curried lamb chops, pg. 63	.0

MID-AFTERNOON

Omelet, pg. 55	2.0
½ cup fresh cantaloupe	6.0

DINNER	Carbohydrates
Steak, grilled or broiled	.0
1 cup cauliflower	5.0

EARLY EVENING

3 eggs, any style	1.2

Total Daily Carbohydrates 32.4

THIRD DAY

BREAKFAST

3 eggs, any style	1.2
Breakfast steak	.0
½ cup fresh cantaloupe	6.0

MID-MORNING

Stuffed tomatoes, pg. 56	8.0
1 hard boiled egg	trace

LUNCH

Stuffed burger, pg. 57	trace

MID-MORNING

Omelet, pg. 55	2.0

DINNER

Lamb steak marinade, pg. 63	.0
½ cup gingered carrots, pg. 55	5.0
Dinner salad	5.0

EARLY EVENING

3 eggs, any style	1.2

Total Daily Carbohydrates 31.4

FOURTH DAY

BREAKFAST

3 eggs, any style	1.2
Cube steak	.0
1 fresh peach	12.0

MID-MORNING

Shrimp salad, pg. 53	5.0

LUNCH

Stuffed burger, pg. 57	trace

MID-AFTERNOON

Omelet, pg. 55	2.0
½ cup fresh cantaloupe	6.0

DINNER

Liver, pg. 60	trace
½ cup asparagus, pg. 56	4.0

EARLY EVENING	Carbohydrates
3 eggs, any style	1.2

Total Daily Carbohydrates 31.4

FIFTH DAY

BREAKFAST
3 eggs, any style	1.2
Baked chicken breast	.0
1 cup fresh strawberries	12.0

MID-MORNING
Fresh mushroom salad, pg. 53	5.0

LUNCH
Garlic lamb steaks, pg. 63	.0
2 stuffed eggs, pg. 52	trace

MID-AFTERNOON
Omelet, pg. 55	2.0
½ cup fresh cantaloupe	6.0

DINNER
Ribbon meatloaf, pg. 59	trace
1 cup skillet zucchini, pg. 55	4.0

EARLY EVENING
3 eggs, any style	1.2

Total Daily Carbohydrates 31.0

NOTE: On Saturday and Sunday, repeat the weekday menu of your choice.

2nd WEEK

FIRST DAY

BREAKFAST
3 eggs, any style	1.2
Cold shrimp and lemon	trace
½ cup fresh cantaloupe	6.0

MID-MORNING
Tuna salad, pg. 53	5.0

LUNCH
Baked Italian chicken, pg. 61	.0

MID-AFTERNOON
Omelet, pg. 55	2.0

DINNER	Carbohydrates
Baked fish, pg. 62	.0
Dinner salad	5.0

EARLY EVENING
3 eggs, any style	1.2

Total Daily Carbohydrates 20.4

SECOND DAY

BREAKFAST
3 eggs, any style	1.2
Baked chicken breast	.0
½ cup fresh cantaloupe	6.0

MID-MORNING
Shrimp salad, pg. 53	5.0

LUNCH
Cornish hen, pg. 61	3.0

MID-AFTERNOON
Omelet, pg. 55	2.0

DINNER
Tarragon chicken in wine, pg. 61	trace
Cheese broiled tomatoes, pg. 56	3.0

EARLY EVENING
3 eggs, any style	1.2

Total Daily Carbohydrates 21.4

THIRD DAY

BREAKFAST
3 eggs, any style	1.2
Chicken breast with Swiss cheese	trace
½ cup fresh cantaloupe	6.0

MID-MORNING
Turkey salad, pg. 53	5.0

LUNCH
Parmesan chicken, pg. 61	trace
2 stuffed eggs, pg. 52	trace

MID-AFTERNOON
Omelet, pg. 55	2.0

DINNER
Cod and cheese sauce, pg. 62	trace
1 cup cheese broiled asparagus, pg. 56	6.0

EARLY EVENING	Carbohydrates
3 eggs, any style	1.2

Total Daily Carbohydrates 21.4

FOURTH DAY

BREAKFAST

3 eggs, any style	1.2
Cold chicken	.0
½ cup fresh cantaloupe	6.0

MID-MORNING

Tuna salad, pg. 53	5.0

LUNCH

Sliced turkey	.0
2 stuffed eggs, pg. 52	trace

MID-AFTERNOON

Omelet, pg. 55	2.0

DINNER

Marinated salmon steaks, pg. 62	.0
1 cup seasoned green beans, pg. 56	4.0

EARLY EVENING

3 eggs, any style	1.2

Total Daily Carbohydrates 19.4

FIFTH DAY

BREAKFAST

3 eggs, any style	1.2
Flaked tuna with lemon	trace
½ cup fresh cantaloupe	6.0

MID-MORNING

Turkey salad, pg. 53	5.0

LUNCH

Baked fish piquant, pg. 62	.0
2 stuffed eggs, pg. 52	trace

MID-AFTERNOON

Omelet, pg. 55	2.0

DINNER

Boiled shrimp with lemon butter pg. 62	trace
Lite salad, pg. 53	3.0
½ cup seasoned green beans, pg. 56	2.0

EARLY EVENING	Carbohydrates
3 eggs, any style	1.2

Total Daily Carbohydrates 20.4

NOTE: On Saturday and Sunday, repeat the weekday menu of your choice.

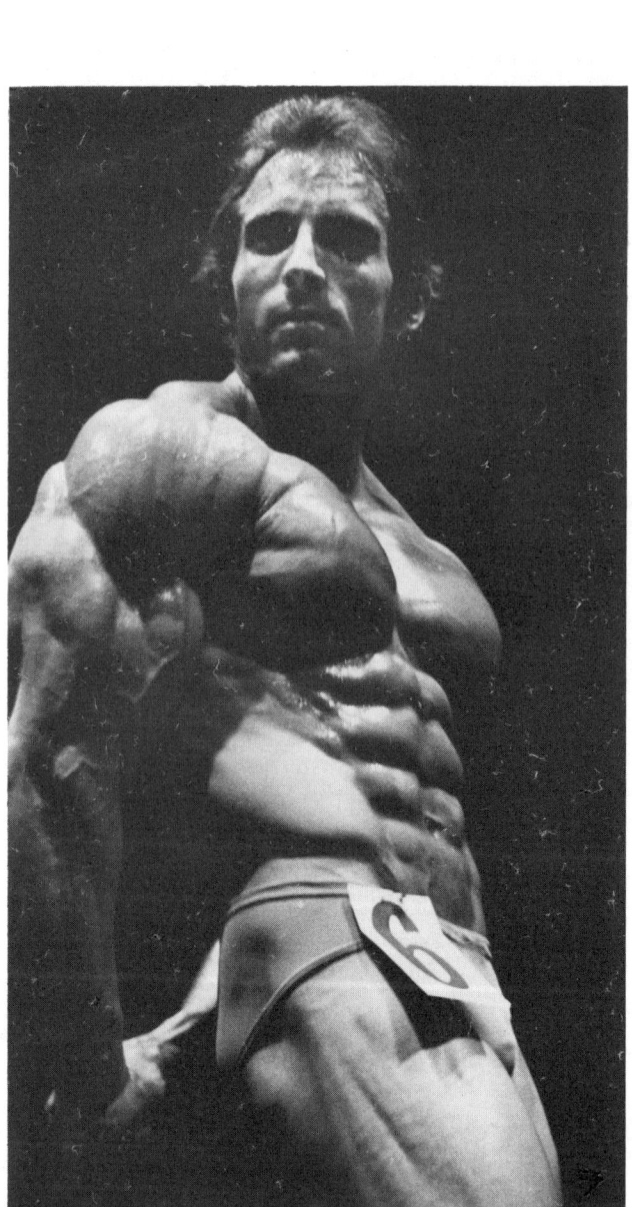

**PAT NEVE
MR. AMERICA
1976**

THE FINAL WEEK

During the final week of training on the *Countdown Diet*, the carbohydrates are reduced to about 10 grams a day. Since carbohydrates are largely responsible for supplying the body with fuel for energy, the intensity of the workouts will definitely be effected. Yet along with the cut-back in carbohydrates there is, among many top bodybuilders, a technique of reducing the workouts too.

Often the physique gets used to hard training and reaches a certain point in its peak where mysteriously it quits responding. At this point many bodybuilders simply start coasting through the workouts. This coasting technique enables the body to replenish and rebuild, and avoids the famous "overtraining syndrome."

The idea this last week is to get a fast, light, total body workout, enough to get a good pump to each muscle group. Some bodybuilders might find it necessary to add 10 to 20 extra grams of carbohydrates just prior to or during the workout.

Some iced-tea with 1 to 2 teaspoons of fructose works well. Also raw fruits, nuts and sunflower seeds are excellent. Be sure the nuts and seeds are raw and unsalted. Also an increase in desiccated liver will miracuously help fight fatigue. During the final week before competition, Pat takes up to 20 liver tablets a day and swears by its effectiveness in fighting the fatigue.

FIRST DAY

BREAKFAST	Carbohydrates
3 eggs, any style	1.2
Tuna with lemon juice	trace
¼ cup fresh cantaloupe	3.0

MID-MORNING	
4 stuffed eggs, pg. 53	1.0

LUNCH	
Baked Italian chicken, pg. 61	trace
Sliced cheese	trace

MID-AFTERNOON	
Omelet, pg. 55	2.0

DINNER	Carbohydrates
Barbecued fish, pg. 62	.0
2 slices fresh tomatoes	1.0

EARLY EVENING	
3 eggs, any style	1.2

Total Daily Carbohydrates 9.4

SECOND DAY

BREAKFAST	
3 eggs, any style	1.2
Baked chicken breast	.0
¼ cup fresh cantaloupe	3.0

MID-MORNING	
Flaked tuna with lemon juice	trace
1 hard boiled egg	trace

LUNCH	
Fish with wine and tomatoes, pg. 63	trace

MID-AFTERNOON	
Omelet, pg. 55	2.0

DINNER	
Parmesan chicken, pg. 61	trace
½ cup seasoned green beans	3.0

EARLY EVENING	
3 eggs, any style	1.2

Total Daily Carbohydrates 10.4

THIRD DAY

BREAKFAST	
3 eggs, any style	1.2
Cold shrimp	.0
¼ cup fresh cantaloupe	3.0

MID-MORNING	
Turkey Oscar, pg. 60	trace
1 hard boiled egg	trace

LUNCH	
Cod and cheese sauce, pg. 62	trace

MID-AFTERNOON	
Omelet, pg. 55	2.0

DINNER	
Tarragon chicken in wine, pg. 61	trace
½ cup spinach	3.0

EARLY EVENING	Carbohydrates
3 eggs, any style	1.2

Total Daily Carbohydrates 10.4

FOURTH DAY

BREAKFAST

	Carbohydrates
3 eggs, any style	1.2
Sliced turkey	.0
¼ cup fresh canteloupe	3.0

MID-MORNING

Cold shrimp with lemon juice	trace
2 stuffed eggs, pg. 52	trace

LUNCH

Baked Italian chicken, pg. 61	.0

DINNER

Baked fish, pg. 62	.0
½ cup seasoned green beans	3.0

EARLY EVENING

3 eggs, any style	1.2

Total Daily Carbohydrates 10.4

FIFTH DAY

BREAKFAST

	Carbohydrates
3 eggs, any style	1.2
Baked chicken breast	.0
¼ cup fresh canteloupe	3.0

MID-MORNING

Flaked salmon with lemon juice	trace
2 stuffed eggs, pg. 52	trace

LUNCH

Roast turkey	.0
Sliced cheese	trace

MID-AFTERNOON

Omelet, pg. 55	2.0

DINNER

Red Snapper Almondine	trace
1 cup skillet zucchini, pg. 55	4.0

EARLY EVENING

3 eggs, any style	1.2

Total Daily Carbohydrates 11.4

NOTE: On Saturday and Sunday, repeat the weekday menu of your choice.

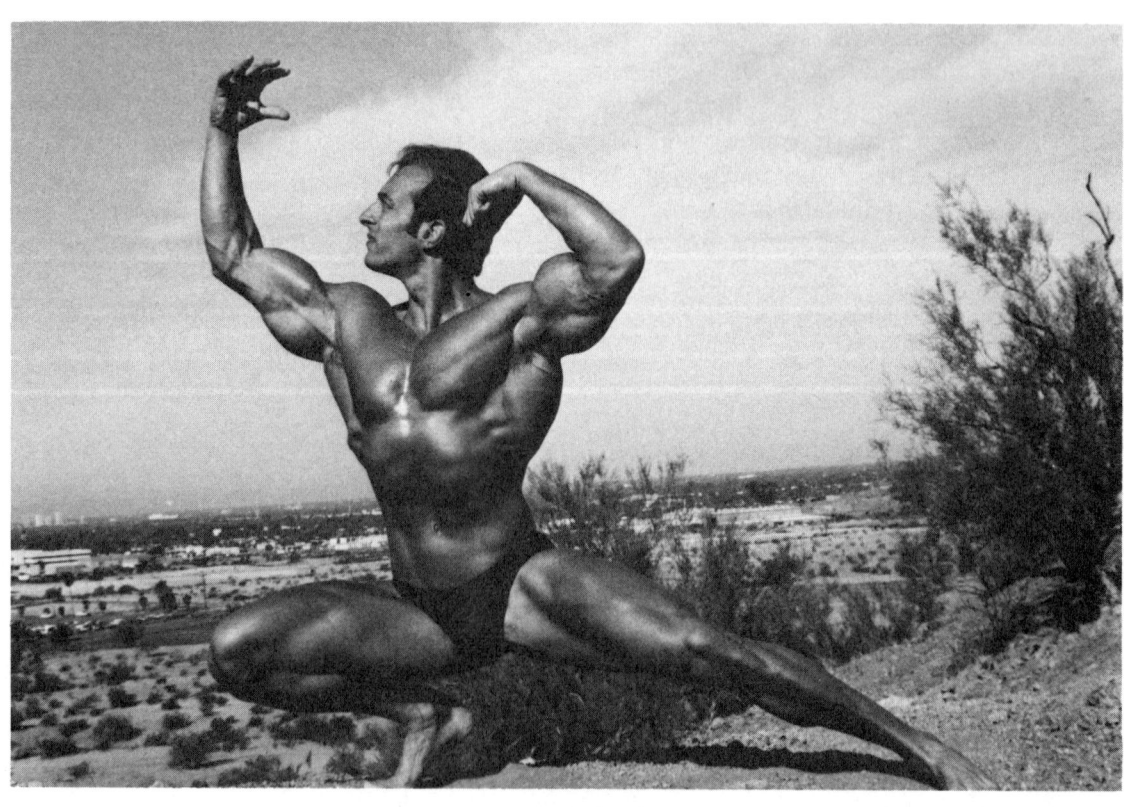

PAT, AGE 31

VII
WOMEN'S BODYBUILDING and 14-DAY MENU PLAN

In the 1970's, a whole new dimension in the sport of bodybuilding opened up — bodybuilding by women. The Equal Rights movement during this decade allowed women to pursue and experience many areas once open only to men. Society quickly accepted women truckdrivers, construction workers, heavy machinery operators, and mechanics. For years, women athletes have proven themselves fit and able to compete in athletic events.

But we were all amazed to see women's powerlifting get off the ground, quite successfully, I might add. Woman have proven their strength and ability, pound for pound; again achieving goals that were once only allowed to men. In women's quest for further achievements, the sport of bodybuilding was no exception.

In June of 1979 the first World Women's Bodybuilding Championships were staged on the West Coast, in which the first lady of women's bodybuilding was crowned — Lisa Lyon. I didn't see the contest, but Pat did. When he told me about it, I have to admit I was not enthusiastic about women's ability or credibility in bodybuilding. I **did** see Lisa guest-pose at the **1979 Mr. Olympia** contest, and I was totally impressed with her performance. She displayed a fine degree of muscle development, with very good definition, and topped it all with a beautiful posing routine. Since then, I have seen many impressive women bodybuilders and gained a new understanding and respect of their achievements. Because of the bold efforts of those dedicated women, another door has been unlocked, and women's bodybuilding has established its credibility.

There must have been hundreds of girls across the country just waiting for such an opportunity because the response to women's bodybuilding was overwhelming. Because of this response, my husband Pat, and his good friend and associate, Fred Scelzo, decided to hold Phoenix's first women's bodybuilding competition along with their annual **Mr. Phoenix Bodybuilding Championships.** The interest was very strong, yet because the sport was new, many girls found themselves lacking the proper coaching and counseling in the various requirements of training, diet, and presentation.

So Pat set up a women's bodybuilding clinic with Kay Baxter, **Women's National Physique Champion and Miss Southwest.** The clinic was designed to help educate would-be women competiors in the requirements of women's bodybuilding. In helping to counsel these girls on training and diet, Pat and I recognized the need for individual diet techniques for women's bodybuilding. We were able to observe Kay Baxter's personal diet techniques and apply many of those principles along with our own to aid in our gym for the women's bodybuilding competition. The results were very encouraging. We subsequently polished these diet techniques as a basis for competitive women's bodybuilding.

As the sport matures, so will the various diet techniques, but we feel the diet presented here is a sound approach to training requirements for today's female competition.

THE WOMEN'S BODYBUILDING DIET

Basically, the same principles on diet apply to both men and women bodybuilders, with the emphasis on high protein and lower carbohydrates. But female competitors do not require the same amount of calories as men, because they are not maintaining the same degree of muscle mass.

Instead of six meals a day, we found four, much smaller meals, were better suited to women's needs. One important factor in women's physiques was made very clear to us during the final weeks before our competition. They needed to lose a lot more weight than anticipated to best display their muscular development. We found the *Women's Bodybuilding Diet* proved most effective when began 4 to 6 weeks before competition. In producing a leaner look, the women were able to maintain their individual degree of muscle-size and still acquire definition.

WOMEN'S BODYBUILDING DIET FORMAT

Weeks Prior to Competition	Meal Make-up	Daily Carbohydrates
4 - 6 weeks	Eggs Fowl & Fish Cheese Fruits Vegetables	Should remain under 30 grams

Of course, a lot depends on the individual's stage of muscle development and the intensity of the workouts, but we feel the *Women's Bodybuilding Diet* is an excellent format to follow in the sport of Women's Bodybuilding.

THE MENUS

FIRST DAY   Carbohydrates

BREAKFAST 8:00 a.m.

1 egg, any style	trace
½ cup fresh or unsw. frozen strawberries	6

MID-MORNING 11:00 a.m.

4 - Egg toppers, pg. 51	1

LUNCH 2:00 p.m.

1 stuffed tomato, pg. 56 (using tuna or cooked chicken for filling)	5
½ cup fresh or unsw. frozen strawberries	6

DINNER 6:00 p.m.

Lite salad, pg. 53	5
2 pc. stuffed celery, pg. 52	3

Total Daily Carbohydrates 26

SECOND DAY   Carbohydrates

BREAKFAST 8:00 a.m.

1 egg, any style	trace
½ med. fresh peach	6

MID-MORNING 11:00 a.m.

½ cup sliced cucumber	2
2 stuffed eggs, pg. 52	trace

LUNCH 2:00 p.m.

1 serving chicken and mushrooms, pg. 61	trace
½ med. fresh peach	6

DINNER 6:00 p.m.

1 cup raw vegetable soup, pg. 52	5
2 oz. cheese	1

Total Daily Carbohydrates 20

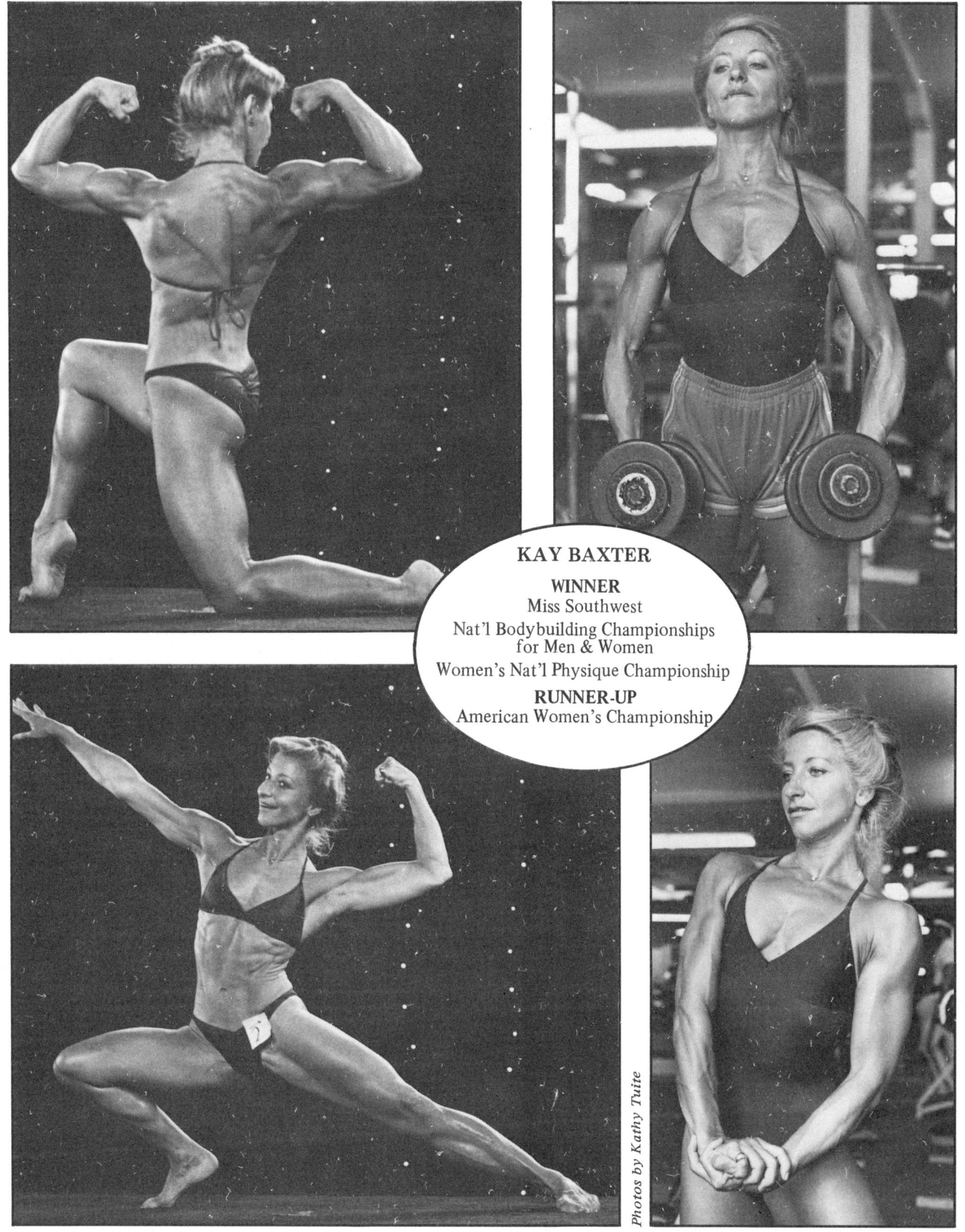

KAY BAXTER

WINNER
Miss Southwest
Nat'l Bodybuilding Championships for Men & Women
Women's Nat'l Physique Championship

RUNNER-UP
American Women's Championship

Photos by Kathy Tuite

THIRD DAY

	Carbohydrates
BREAKFAST 8:00 a.m.	
1 egg, any style	trace
½ cup fresh or unsw. frozen strawberries	6
MID-MORNING 11:00 a.m.	
2 oz. cheese	1
½ raw carrot	2
LUNCH 2:00 p.m.	
1 pc. Turkey Oscar, pg. 60	trace
½ med. fresh peach or unsw. frozen	6
DINNER 6:00 p.m.	
Lite salad, pg. 53	5
1 hard boiled egg	trace

Total Daily Carbohydrates 20

FOURTH DAY

	Carbohydrates
BREAKFAST 8:00 a.m.	
1 egg, any style	trace
½ cup fresh or unsw. frozen strawberries	6
MID-MORNING 11:00 a.m.	
2 pc. stuffed celery, pg. 52	3
LUNCH 2:00 p.m.	
Flaked Salmon with lemon juice	trace
½ cup fresh or unsw. frozen strawberries	6
DINNER 6:00 p.m.	
Lite salad, pg. 53	5
1 hard boiled egg	trace

Total Daily Carbohydrates 20

FIFTH DAY

	Carbohydrates
BREAKFAST 8:00 a.m.	
1 egg, any style	trace
½ med. fresh peach or unsw. frozen	6
MID-MORNING 11:00 a.m.	
2 oz. cheese	1
½ raw carrot	2
LUNCH 2:00 p.m.	
1 pc. Turkey Oscar, pg. 60	trace
½ med. fresh peach or unsw. frozen	6
DINNER 6:00 p.m.	
1 cup raw vegetable soup, pg. 52	5
1 hard boiled egg	trace

Total Daily Carbohydrates 20

SIXTH DAY

	Carbohydrates
BREAKFAST 8:00 a.m.	
1 egg, any style	trace
½ cup fresh or frozen honeydew melon	6
MID-MORNING 11:00 a.m.	
2 stuffed eggs, pg. 52	trace
2 oz. cheese	1
LUNCH 2:00 p.m.	
1 cup Shrimp Salad, pg. 53	5
½ cup fresh honeydew melon	6
DINNER Before 6:00 p.m.	
Lite salad, pg. 53	3
1 small sliced tomato	4

Total Daily Carbohydrates 25

SEVENTH DAY

	Carbohydrates
BREAKFAST 8:00 a.m.	
1 egg, any style	trace
½ cup fresh or unsw. frozen strawberries	6
MID-MORNING 11:00 a.m.	
2 stuffed eggs, pg. 52	trace
2 pcs. stuffed celery	3
LUNCH 2:00 p.m.	
1 cup Turkey Salad, pg. 53	5
½ cup fresh or frozen strawberries	6
DINNER Before 6:00 p.m.	
Lite salad, pg. 53	3
½ cup sliced cucumber	2

Total Daily Carbohydrates 26

JOCELYN FERBIAC

SANDY HARPER

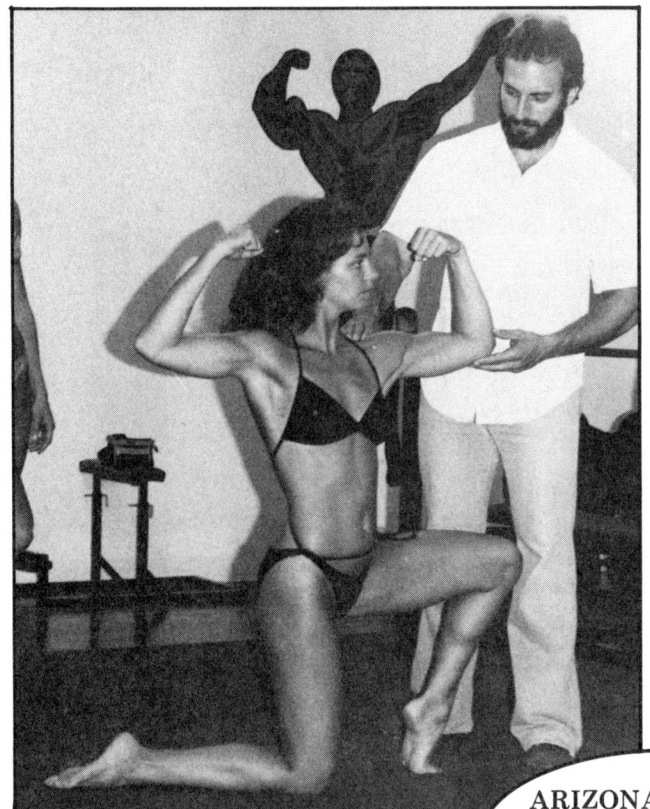
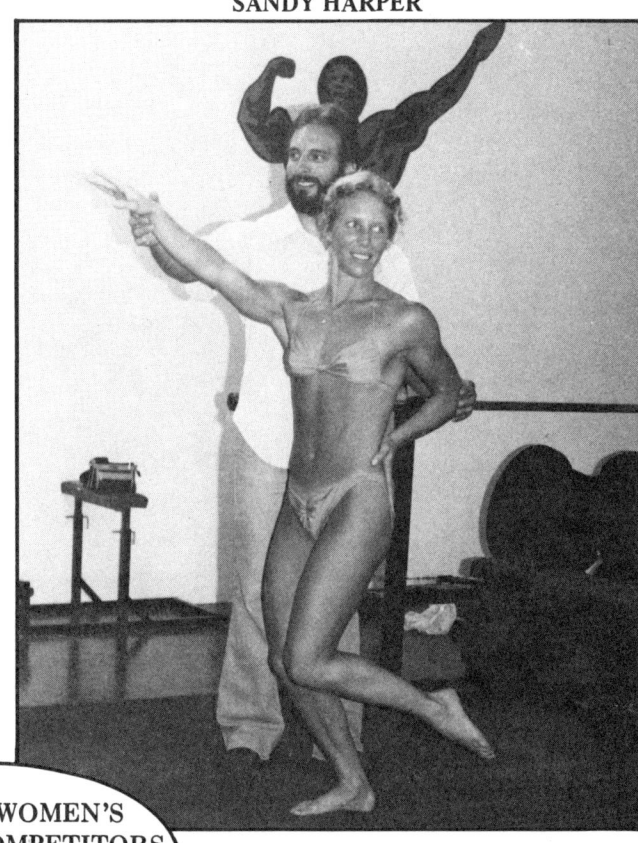

ARIZONA WOMEN'S PHYSIQUE COMPETITORS BEING TRAINED BY PAT NEVE

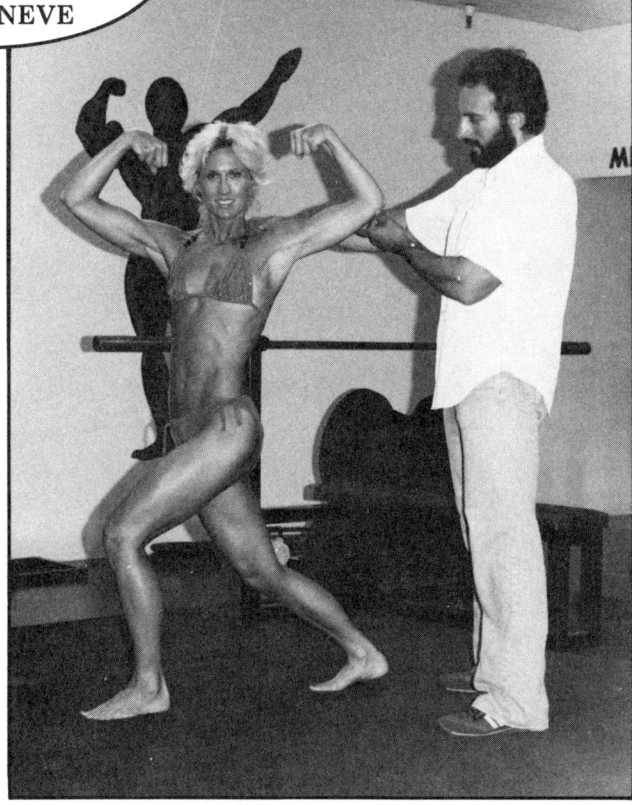

CONNIE SHAKLEFORD

CONNIE SHAKLEFORD

EIGHTH DAY   Carbohydrates

    BREAKFAST 8:00 a.m.

    1 egg, any style   trace
    ½ cup fresh or frozen canteloupe   6

    MID-MORNING 11:00 a.m.

    1 small sliced tomato   4
    2 pcs. stuffed celery, pg. 52   3

    LUNCH 2:00 p.m.

    1 cup tuna salad, pg. 53   5
    ½ cup fresh or frozen canteloupe   6

    DINNER Before 6:00 p.m.

    Small dinner salad with vinegar &
      oil or lemon juice   5
    1 hard boiled egg   trace

Total Daily Carbohydrates 29

NINTH DAY

    BREAKFAST 8:00 a.m.

    1 egg, any style   trace
    ½ cup fresh or frozen canteloupe   6

    MID-MORNING 11:00 a.m.

    1 small sliced tomato   4
    1 hard cooked egg   trace

    LUNCH 2:00 p.m.

    3" wedge Quiche, pg. 54   5
    ½ cup fresh or frozen canteloupe   6

    DINNER 6:00 p.m.

    Lite salad, pg. 53   5
    ½ sliced fresh cucumber   2

Total Daily Carbohydrates 28

TENTH DAY

    BREAKFAST 8:00 a.m.

    1 egg, any style   trace
    ½ cup fresh or frozen honeydew
      melon   6

    MID-MORNING 11:00 a.m.

    2 pcs. stuffed celery   3
    2 oz. cheese   1

    LUNCH 2:00 p.m.

    5 med. cooked shrimp w/lemon
      pg. 62   trace
    ½ cup fresh or frozen honeydew
      melon   6

    DINNER 6:00 p.m.   Carbohydrates

    Lite salad, pg. 53   5
    1 hard boiled egg   trace

Total Daily Carbohydrates 21

ELEVENTH DAY

    BREAKFAST 8:00 a.m.

    1 egg, any style   trace
    ½ cup fresh or unsw. frozen
      strawberries   6

    MID-MORNING 11:00 a.m.

    2 stuffed eggs, pg. 52   trace
    2 oz. cheese   1

    LUNCH 2:00 p.m.

    1 serving Baked Fish, Piquant, pg. 62   trace
    ½ cup fresh or unsw. frozen
      strawberries   6

    DINNER 6:00 p.m.

    Lite salad, pg. 53   5
    ½ raw carrot   2

Total Daily Carbohydrates 20

TWELFTH DAY

    BREAKFAST 8:00 a.m.

    1 egg, any style   trace
    ½ med. peach or unsw. frozen   6

    MID-MORNING 11:00 a.m.

    1 hard cooked egg   trace
    2 pcs. stuffed celery, pg. 52   3

    LUNCH 2:00 p.m.

    1 serving Tropical Chicken, pg. 61   trace
    ½ med. peach or unsw. frozen   6

    DINNER 6:00 p.m.

    Lite salad, pg. 53   5
    2 oz. cheese   1

Total Daily Carbohydrates 21

THIRTEENTH DAY

    BREAKFAST 8:00 a.m.

    1 egg, any style   trace
    ½ cup fresh or frozen canteloupe   6

    MID-MORNING 11:00 a.m.

    2 pcs. stuffed celery, pg. 52   3
    2 oz. cheese   1

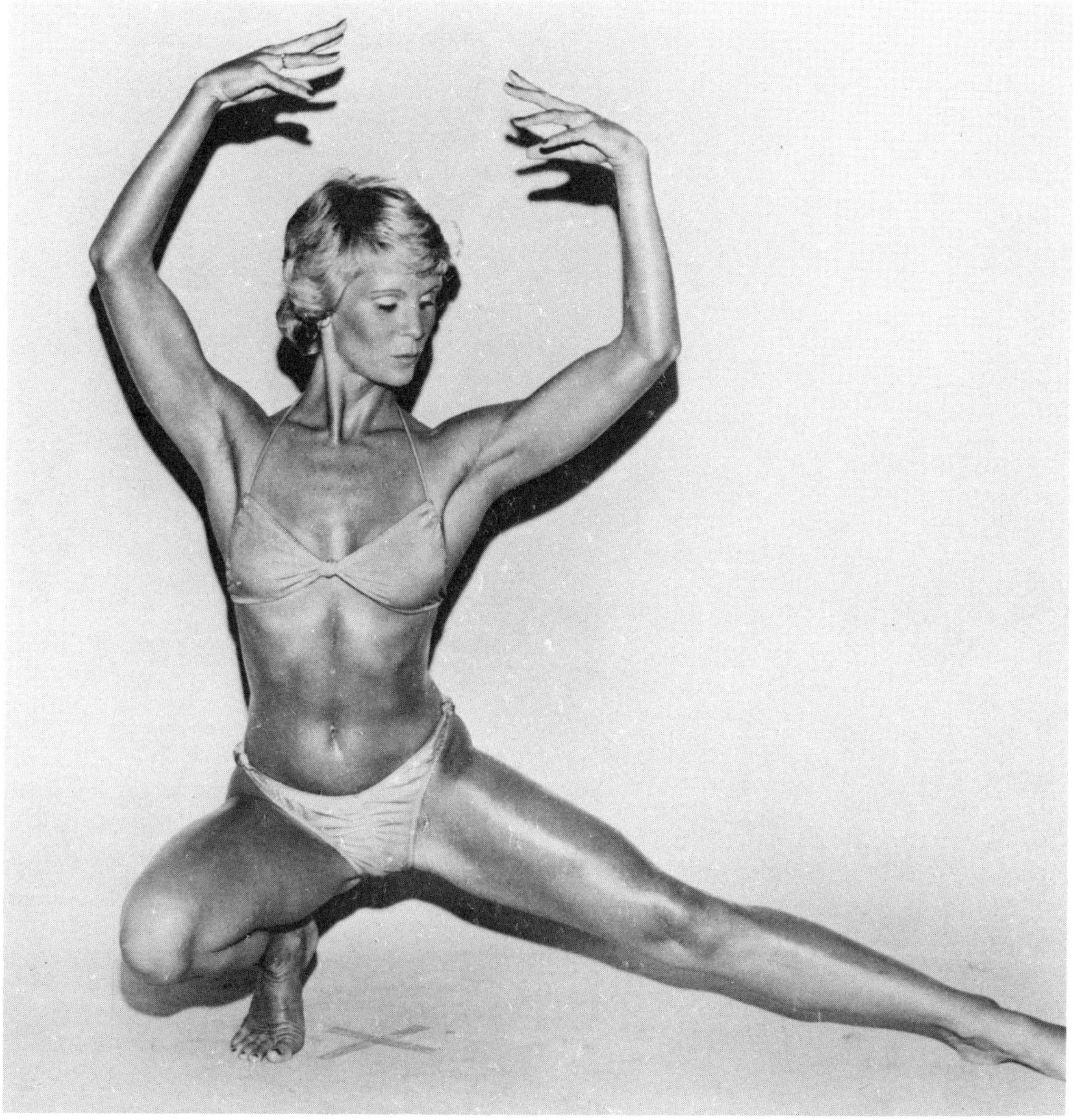

SUSAN BRESSLER
MISS SUN COAST / MISS GOLD COAST

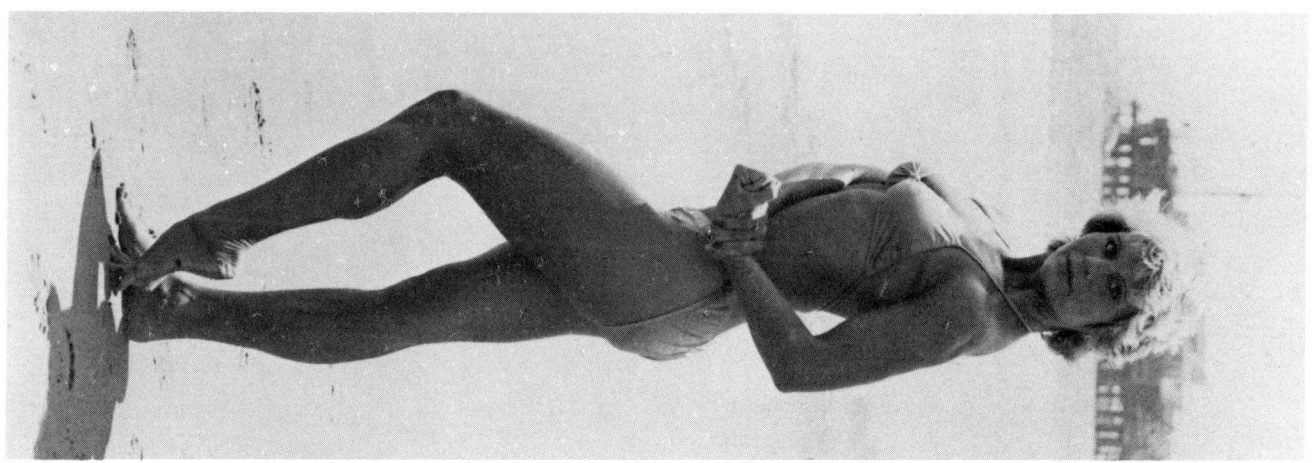

	Carbohydrates
LUNCH 2:00 p.m.	
1 serving Parmesan Chicken, pg. 61	trace
½ cup fresh or frozen canteloupe	6
DINNER 6:00 p.m.	
Lite salad, pg. 53	5
2 stuffed eggs, pg. 52	trace

Total Daily Carbohydrates 21

FOURTEENTH DAY

BREAKFAST 8:00 a.m.	
1 egg, any style	trace
½ cup fresh or unsw. frozen strawberries	6
MID-MORNING 11:00 a.m.	
2 stuffed eggs, pg. 52	trace
½ raw carrot	2
LUNCH 2:00 p.m.	
1 serving Cod & Cheese Sauce, pg. 62	trace
½ cup fresh or unsw. frozen strawberries	6
DINNER 6:00 p.m.	
Lite salad, pg. 53	5
1 small sliced tomato	4

Total Daily Carbohydrates 23

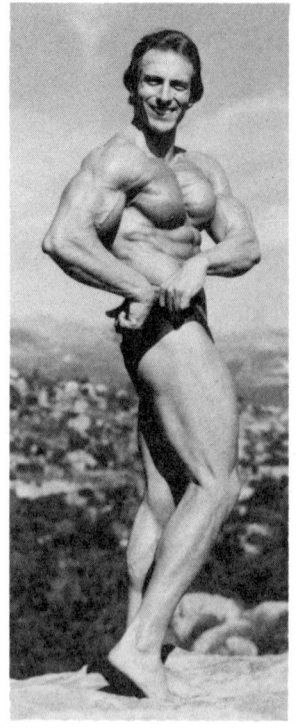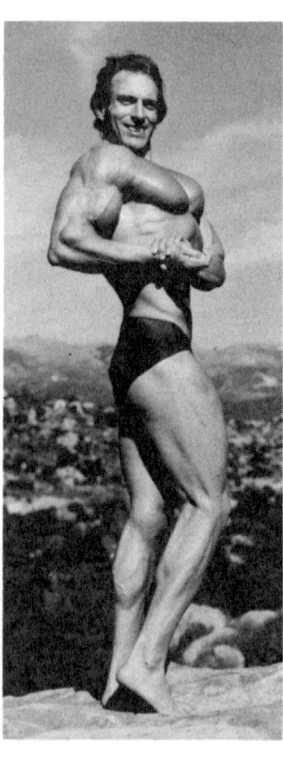

PAT NEVE 1980

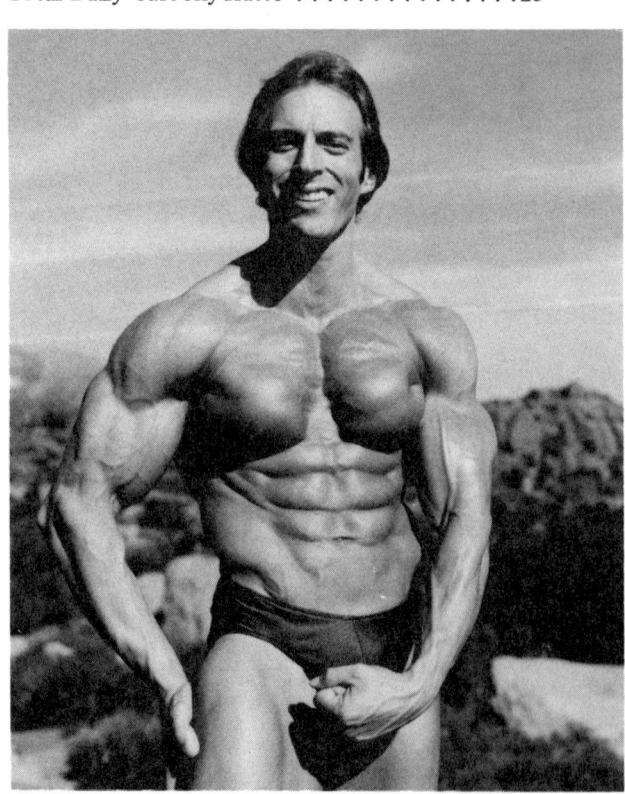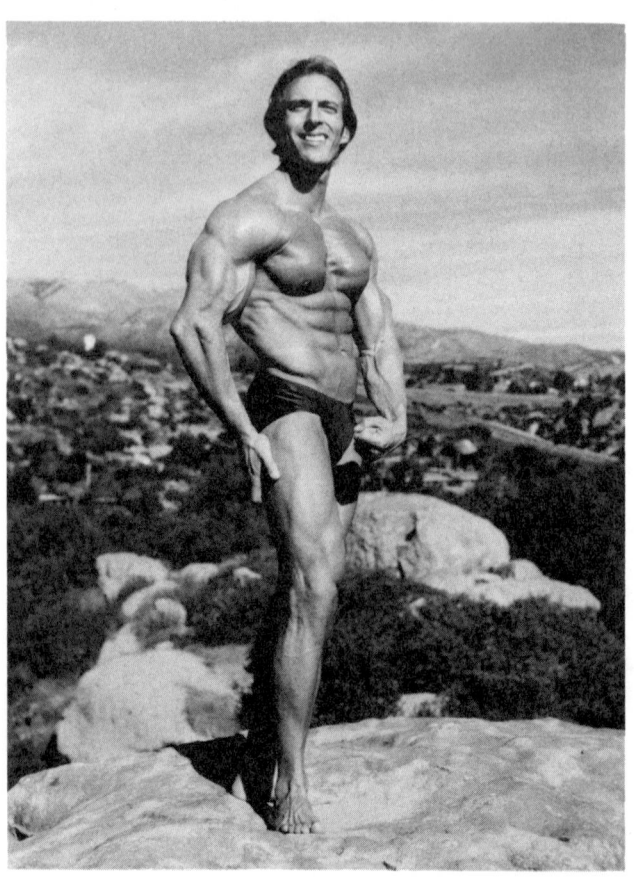

VIII
THE LOW CARBOHYDRATE DIET COOKBOOK

The low carbohydrate diet is more than just an all-out attack on carbohydrates. It is, rather, the role carbohydrates play in blood sugar levels that make them an important factor in a weight loss program. Actually it is the reduction in calories that cause the loss in body weight. By limiting the amount and the type of carbohydrates in your diet, you will automatically cut down on many of the high starch, high calorie foods. At the same time, you will produce a lower and safer blood sugar level.

Carbohydrates serve some important nutritional needs of the body and they should not be completely removed from your daily diet. The low carbohydrate diet in this book does not suggest eliminating carbohydrates altogether. I agree with many experts that the average American consumes far more carbohydrates than necessary.

Each nutrient — carbohydrates, calories, fat and protein — works in conjunction with the others, and the complete elimination of one would be a mistake. It is the balancing of these nutrients to complement each other that becomes the objective. Some refer to it as the Gestalt Nutrition Plan — treating the whole being rather than isolating one area.

It is this balancing that suggests a reduction in the amount and type of carbohydrates. There are two types of carbohydrates: refined and unrefined. The refined carbohydrates, such as candy, cake and colas, are usually higher in refined sugars (sucrose) and drastically raise the blood sugar level for a short period of time. This causes the pancreas to over-react and produce too much insulin, which eventually can cause a reverse condition in the form of low blood sugar or hypoglycemia.

Also, refined carbohydrates do not stay with you as long, and they leave you feeling hungry again shortly after eating. In the long run, unrefined carbohydrates have much more staying power. Furthermore, refined carbohydrates lack nutritional value, the vitamins, mineral and enzymes vital for proper biochemical action of all nutrients.

On the other hand, unrefined carbohydrates such as fruits, vegetables and whole grains, produce a slower, safer insulin reaction, and have a better effect on blood sugar. They contain those vitamins, minerals and enzymes vital in metabolizing calories.

The recipes in *The Low Carbohydrate Cook Book* that follows are designed to reduce the total caloric intake by limiting the amount and kind of carbohydrates. It also attempts to eliminate many refined foods (to a reasonable degree) and balance the overall intake of protein, fats and carbohydrates.

APPETIZERS

EGG TOPPERS
Slice an unpeeled zucchini (Italian squash) in ½ inch slices. Top with a slice of hard-cooked egg; sprinkle with some Spike seasoning and place a small square of cheese on top of each egg slice. Place under a broiler until the cheese starts to melt. Serve warm.

BROILED ZUCCHINI CHIPS
Slice unpeeled zucchini in ½ inch slices. Toss them in a plastic bag with 1/3 cup of grated Parmesan cheese. Place each zucchini slice on a cookie sheet sprayed with non-stick spray. Top with an additional ½ teaspoon of Parmesan cheese

and pat lightly. Broil for 3 to 5 minutes until golden brown. Remove with pancake turner and serve warm.

STUFFED EGGS, TURKEY OR CHICKEN
Chop one cup of cooked chicken or turkey very fine; or put it through a meat grinder. Add ½ teaspoon of Spike seasoning; 1 tablespoon of diced black olives; 1 tablespoon of finely diced celery; 1 tablespoon of finely diced fresh tomatoes; ¼ cup of fine grated Swiss cheese (optional). Stir in enough imitation mayonnaise to moisten. Fill cooked egg whites. Garnish with parsley.

STUFFED EGGS, LOBSTER, CRABMEAT, TUNA OR SALMON
Remove cartilage from six ½ oz. cans of crabmeat or lobster, or drain liquid from the same amount of tuna or salmon. Rinse thoroughly. Remove skin from salmon. Flake fish fine. Add ½ cup finely chopped celery; 2 tablespoons chopped green pepper, and 1/4 cup cheese grated fine (optional). Season with Spike seasoning and pepper to taste. Add 1½ teaspoons of lemon juice to tuna or salmon. Stir in enough imitation mayonnaise to moisten, and fill hard-cooked egg whites. Garnish with olive slices.
Use the leftover egg yolks to garnish salads and vegetables.

GUACAMOLE
Peel three ripe avocados and remove seeds. Put them in a bowl and mash with a potato masher. Add ¼ cup of diced fresh tomatoes; 2 or 3 chopped green onions (include some dark green stalk); 1 minced fresh garlic clove; 1 teaspoon of crushed red chili pepper; 1 teaspoon of vinegar; ½ teaspoon of oregano; 2 tablespoons of lemon juice; a dash of tabasco; 1 Jalapeno pepper, minced (optional); and stir. Cover and chill for one hour.

GUACAMOLE STUFFED CELERY
Wash celery stalks and cut off the leafy tops. Cut in finger-length pieces and stuff with guacamole. Sprinkle with grated Monterey Jack or Cheddar cheese.

Spike is a natural vegetable seasoning.

BROILED MUSHROOMS AND BACON
Wash and remove stems from large fresh mushrooms. Put 1 drop of lemon juice in each cap and wrap in ½ slice of bacon, fastening with a toothpick. Put wrapped mushrooms on a rack and broil until they are tender and the bacon is crisp. Turn twice during broiling.

SOUPS

RAW VEGETABLE SOUP
Place diced summer zucchini squash, carrots, cabbage and celery in a blender and blend until creamy. Add some sauteed onions, and heat just to serving temperature (cooking destroys many vitamins and minerals in food). Sprinkle with some Spike seasoning and grated Parmesan cheese, and serve.

ONION SOUP
Brown three large, sliced onions slowly in butter. Add 1/3 cup of sliced green onions; 4 tablespoons of butter; 5 cups of bouillon; ½ cup of grated Parmesan cheese; pepper to taste; and let simmer for 30 minutes. To serve, place a thin slice of Provelone cheese on top of each hot serving.

SPICY MEATBALL SOUP
3 cups prepared Instant Beef Boullion (with no salt added); ¼ cup chopped green chilies; ¼ cup chopped green onion, with stalk; 1 small diced tomato; 1/8 teaspoon cumin; garlic powder and pepper to taste; 6 meatballs, (pg.00)
Simmer all ingredients, covered, for 15 - 20 minutes. Top each serving with 1 tablespoon grated Monterey Jack cheese.

SALADS

HOT SPINACH SALAD
Wash and remove the stems from 8 ounces of fresh spinach, and dry the leaves. Tear the leaves into bite-size pieces; add 2 slices of crisply cooked crumbled bacon; heat 1/3 cup vinegar and oil dressing; toss bacon and spinach; pour on heated dressing and toss again.

LITE SALAD

Tear bite-sized pieces of lettuce and ¼ cup of raw bean sprouts, toss with fresh or concentrated lemon juice and sugar substitute. Garnish with one thin slice of tomato.

TUNA SALAD

1 - 9 ¼ oz. can water-packed tuna, drained
½ cup shredded longhorn cheese
1 cup shredded Iceberg lettuce
2 hard-boiled eggs, chopped
½ cup of tomatoes, diced
¼ cup black olives, chopped

Toss all ingredients together with imitation mayonnaise, and serve.

SHRIMP SALAD

12 oz. small fresh shrimp, de-veined or:
2 - 6oz. pkgs. frozen, thawed and rinsed shrimp (Del Monte)
4 hard-boiled eggs, chopped
1 cup of shredded cheese of choice, optional
1 tablespoon pimientos, diced
2 tablespoons imitation mayonnaise, containing no sugar
1 teaspoon lemon juice

Combine first four ingredients; mix mayonnaise and lemon juice; toss salad and mayonnaise dressing, serve on a bed of lettuce sprinkled with paprika.

FRESH MUSHROOM SALAD

½ head Romaine, washed and chilled
½ head Iceberg lettuce, washed/chilled
¼ pound fresh mushrooms, trimmed and sliced
Fancy vinegar and oil dressing

Line salad bowl with Romaine leaves; tear bite-sized pieces of lettuce into bowl; add mushrooms; pour on fancy vinegar and oil dressing and toss.

FRUIT SALAD

½ cup fresh strawberries
½ cup fresh sliced peaches
½ cup fresh bing cherries, pitted
¼ cup fresh red raspberries
2 cups fresh cantaloupe balls
¼ cup walnuts

Mix 1 cup sour cream or plain yogurt and 1 teaspoon fructose. Gently fold in fruits and nuts. Makes eight ½ cup servings; approximately eight carbohydrates each.

PEACH-N-CHEESE SALAD

2/3 cup low-fat creamed cottage cheese
¼ teaspoon cinnamon
1/8 teaspoon cloves
2 tablespoons toasted slivered blanched almonds
4 fresh or unsweetened canned peach halves
Crisp greens

Mix cottage cheese, almonds, cinnamon and cloves. Fill center of peach halves with cheese mixture. Arrange on crisp greens.

HEARTY BEEF SALAD

2 cups roast beef, cooked and cut into slices
1 cup torn Iceberg lettuce
½ cup diced tomatoes
2 hard-boiled eggs, chopped
½ cup cubed Swiss cheese

Dressing: 1 cup imitation mayonnaise; 2 teaspoons dry mustard; 1 teaspoon garlic powder; 3 tablespoons lemon juice; pepper and Spike seasoning.

Arrange salad on platter or toss together in salad bowl. Pour on dressing and serve.

TURKEY SALAD

2 cups cooked and cubed turkey breast
2 hard-boiled eggs, chopped
½ cup diced tomatoes
¼ cup diced celery
½ cup Mozzarella cheese, cubed

Toss all ingredients with imitation mayonnaise containing no sugar.
Serve on a bed of lettuce.

BACON AND EGG SALAD

2 cups hard-boiled eggs, chopped or quartered
4 slices of crisp bacon, crumbled
½ cup shredded longhorn cheese

Toss all ingredients with imitiation mayonnaise containing no sugar.
Serve on a bed of lettuce; garnish with tomato wedges.

DRESSINGS

FANCY VINEGAR AND OIL DRESSING
½ cup salad oil
¼ cup vinegar
¼ cup sliced green onion
¼ cup snipped parsley
1 tablespoon finely chopped green pepper
½ teaspoon fructose
1 teaspoon Spike seasoning
1 teaspoon dry mustard
1/8 teaspoon red pepper

Shake all ingredients in tightly covered jar, and refrigerate. Shake again before serving.
Makes 1 cup.

FRENCH DRESSING
½ cup salad oil
1/3 cup tarragon vinegar
4 teaspoons fructose
1/8 teaspoon dry mustard
1/8 teaspoon black pepper
1 teaspoon paprika
½ teaspoon onion juice

Combine all ingredients and beat with a rotary beater. Chill and shake before serving.

SOUR CREAM DRESSING
1 egg yolk
2 teaspoons vinegar
½ teaspoon dry mustard
3 teaspoons fructose
¼ teaspoon Spike seasoning
Dash of pepper
½ cup sour cream

Beat egg yolk in top of double boiler until thick. Stir in remaining ingredients except sour cream. Place over simmering water and cook, stirring constantly until slightly thickened. Cool and stir in sour cream. Chill thoroughly before serving.

SESAME SALAD DRESSING
1 tablespoon sesame seeds
2 tablespoons of water
2 tablespoons wine vinegar
1½ teaspoons fresh lemon juice
1¼ teaspoons Spike seasoning
½ cup salad oil
¼ teaspoon fructose
1 medium clove garlic, sliced
Dash black pepper
2 teaspoons finely cut parsley

Spread sesame seeds on a shallow pan and toast in 350-degree oven to light tan color. Combine remaining ingredients in jar, add sesame seeds and shake vigorously. Let stand 30 minutes and remove garlic. Cover and refrigerate. Shake well before serving.

LOW CARBOHYDRATE RECIPES

NO-CRUST QUICHE
1 cup skim milk
6 eggs
1 cup grated cheese, any kind
1 teaspoon paprika, nutmeg or cayenne

Beat eggs, skim milk and spice thoroughly. Fold in cheese. Pour mixture into a 9-inch deep dish pie plate sprayed with no-stick vegetable coating. Bake in preheated 350 degree oven for 45 minutes to 1 hour or until knife inserted in center comes out clean.
This will also make 2 standard 8-inch pies.

NO CRUST QUICHE VARIATIONS
#1 ¾ cup diced cooked turkey or chicken
#2 ¾ cup small cocktail shrimp and ½ cup sliced mushrooms
#3 ¼ - ½ cup diced green chilies and ¾ cup cooked ground beef
#4 ¾ cup diced fresh tomato and 2 pcs. cooked crisp bacon, crumbled

BASIC SCRAMBLED EGGS
2 or 3 eggs
¼ teaspoon paprika

Beat eggs and paprika hard with wire wisk or rotary beater. Melt 1 tablespoon butter (or coat with vegetable oil spray) in pre-heated skillet. Pour in eggs and cook over medium heat, pushing gently with rubber spatula from side-to-side until done to taste. Makes 1 serving.

SCRAMBLED EGG VARIATIONS
Add:
- #1 Avocado, green onion and longhorn cheese
- #2 Crumbled bacon and Swiss cheese
- #3 Sour cream or plain yogurt, black olives and cocktail shrimp
- #4 Diced cooked lamb, green pepper and Monterey jack cheese
- #5 Diced cooked chicken and sauteed onion, celery and pinch of sage

BASIC OMELET
2 or 3 eggs, separated
1 tablespoon skim milk

Beat egg yolks and milk together. Whip egg whites until stiff, and gently fold into yolk mixture. Melt 1 tablespoon butter in teflon skillet. Pour in eggs and cook over low heat until set enough to turn, like a pancake. Turn and cook 30 more seconds. Fold omelet in half. Makes 1 serving.

PUFFY OMELET
2 or 3 eggs, separated
1 tablespoon skim milk

Beat egg yolks and milk together. Whip egg whites until stiff, and gently fold into yolk mixture. Melt 1 tablespoon butter in teflon skillet and pour in eggs. Cook over low heat until set and turn like a pancake. Cook 30 seconds longer; fold in half. Makes 1 serving.

OMELET VARIATIONS
Add:
- #1 Sliced leftover meatloaf and cheese
- #2 Cooked shrimp, sauteed in butter, lemon and parsley
- #3 Diced leftover steak or roast and sauteed onion rings
- #4 Sliced leftover Italian meatballs, sauce and Mozarella cheese
- #5 Fresh sliced mushrooms sauteed in butter, parsley and pinch of tarragon

VEGETABLES

GINGERED CARROTS
6 medium carrots, scraped and cut into ½ inch slices
2 teaspoons lemon juice
½ teaspoon ground ginger
Dash pepper
2 tablespoons butter

Put carrots in buttered 1-quart casserole. Mix lemon juice and seasonings; pour over carrots and dot with butter. Cover and bake in pre-heated oven at 400 degrees for 1 hour.

BROCCOLI AND BACON
1 package (10 oz.) frozen broccoli, cut up
2 slices of bacon, diced
½ garlic clove, minced
2 tablespoons cider vinegar
¼ cup grated Parmesan cheese

Cook broccoli according to package directions. Meanwhile, cook bacon and garlic until bacon is crisp. Add vinegar, and heat. Pour sauce over broccoli and sprinkle with Parmesan cheese.

MARINATED CUCUMBERS AND ONIONS
3 cucumbers
1 small red onion
1 cup vinegar
½ cup water
¼ cup chopped parsley
2 tablespoons fructose
¼ teaspoon pepper

Peel and slice cucumbers and onion very thin. Add remaining ingredients. Refrigerate for 2 hours before serving.

SKILLET ZUCCHINI
2 medium zucchini, sliced
2 slices of onion, rings separated
1 small tomato, diced
1 garlic clove, minced
2 tablespoons butter
½ cup grated Parmesan cheese

Melt butter in skillet over medium heat. Add zucchini, onion rings, tomato and garlic. Saute, stirring occasionally, until onion is clear in color. Stir in Parmesan cheese. Serve.

STUFFED TOMATOES
5 medium-sized tomatoes
1 tablespoon butter
1 tablespoon oil
1 small onion, chopped fine
3/4 pound lean ground beef
Pepper to taste

Slice the top off each tomato and save. Spoon out the seeds. Carefully spoon out the pulp and set aside. Place tomatoes upside down to drain. Saute onion in heated oil and butter until transparent. Add meat and cook for 5 minutes, stirring with wooden spoon. Add tomato pulp and pepper. Cook over low heat for 15 minutes. Fill each tomato with meat mixture, mounding meat on top. Replace tomato tops. Place in buttered baking dish and cover with buttered wax paper. Bake in 350 degree oven for 20 minutes. Serve warm.

SEASONED GREEN BEANS
1 - 8¾ oz. can green beans (Del Monte)
3 slices of bacon
1 tablespoon minced onion
Garlic powder
1 teaspoon Spike seasoning
Pepper

Fry bacon in saucepan until it starts to crisp up. Add green beans with liquid and onion. Add garlic powder, Spike and pepper to taste. Simmer 15 minutes.

SPINACH AND BROCCOLI
1½ cups fresh spinach, or 1 package (10 oz.) frozen chopped spinach
1½ cups fresh broccoli, or 1 package (10 oz.) frozen, chopped broccoli
2/3 cup water
1 teaspoon Spike seasoning
1 tablespoon lemon juice

In covered saucepan, heat brocolli, spinach, water and Spike to boiling. Reduce heat; simmer until tender. If using frozen vegetables, follow package directions. Drain, toss with lemon juice.

CHEESE-BROILED ASPARAGUS
Put cooked asparagus spears in shallow baking dish or pie-pan. Sprinkle generously with grated Romano cheese. Put under broiler until heated.

CHEESE TOMATO BROIL
2 large fresh tomatoes
½ pound low-fat creamed cottage cheese
½ cup grated Parmesan cheese
Salt and pepper

Cut each tomato into 3 thick slices. Broil on one side and turn. Mix cheese, salt and pepper to taste. Spread generously on tomato slices and broil until golden brown and bubbly.

STUFFED MUSHROOMS
Remove stems from large fancy muchrooms and chop. Cook 3 slices of bacon until crisp; remove bacon and pour off fat, leaving about 2 tablespoons . Add mushroom stems, 1 onion, chopped fine; and ¼ cup chopped green pepper. Cook until tender. Add ¾ cup grated Parmesan cheese, crumbled bacon, 2 tablespoons chopped parsley, salt and pepper to taste. Stuff mushroom caps. Place in shallow baking dish with small amount of water (about ¼ inch deep). Bake in preheated slow oven at 325 degrees for about 25 minutes. Stuffing fills about 12 large fancy mushroom caps.

SPINACH
1 pound fresh spinach
1 cup boiling water
½ teaspoon Spike seasoning
2 tablespoons butter

Cut away course stems from spinach and discard. Wash spinach thoroughly and drain well. Cut crosswise into 1 inch strips, and bring to boil in saucepan. Cover and boil 6 to 10 minutes. Drain thoroughly. Add melted butter, toss and serve immediately.

CAULIFLOWER WITH CHEESE
Wash fresh cauliflower head and trim base of stalk; discard all large leaves. Separate floweretts. Drop into boiling water and boil gently for 6 to 8 minutes. Remove from water with slotted spoon. Arrange on oven-safe serving platter, and sprinkle with a mixture of shredded Monterey Jack and sharp cheddar cheese. Place under broiler until cheese starts to melt. Serve immediately.

STUFFED PEPPERS

5 green peppers, medium
1 small onion
¼ cup finely chopped parsley
1 cup chopped, cooked, chicken, turkey, veal or ground beef.
2 tablespoons butter
2 ripe tomatoes, medium
½ teaspoon Spike seasoning
Dash pepper
½ cup shredded sharp cheddar cheese

Slice off top of pepper and remove core and seeds. Rinse and drain well. Saute next six ingredients in butter until onion is clear in color. Remove from heat. Stir in cheese, and stuff peppers tightly with filling. Fit peppers snugly in buttered shallow baking pan. Bake in 350 degree oven for 15 to 20 minutes. (Parboiling destroys part of the Vitamin C, and the color quality of peppers).

EVERYTHING YOU EVER WANTED IN A BURGER

BONUS BURGER MIX

3 pounds economy roast
1½ pounds beef heart

Have a butcher grind the roast and heart together like chopped meat. Use this mixture in any recipe calling for hamburger. It is also excellent for disguising other organ meats such as lungs, kidney, liver and brain. They are high in nutrition, and economical as well.

VEGEBURGERS

Lean ground beef
2 tablespoons carrots, shredded
2 tablespoons cabbage, chopped
2 tablespoons summer squash, diced
1 tablespoon parsley, snipped
Spice and pepper to taste

Make six large thin patties with the ground beef. Season with Spike and pepper. Saute vegetables in butter until almost tender. Spoon vegetables equally on 3 patties, leaving ¼ inch clear around the edges. Top with remaining patties; pinching edges to seal. Pan fry, broil or grill to your liking.

CHEESEBURGERS

Lean ground beef
½ cup Ricotta cheese
1 tablespoon grated Parmesan
1 egg
3 slices Mozzarella cheese
1 teaspoon fresh parsley, chopped
Spike and pepper to taste
¾ cup Italian sauce

Make 6 thin patties. Sprinkle with Spike and pepper. Mix Ricotta, egg, Parmesan and parsley. Spoon cheese mixture on 3 patties. Top with a slice of Mozzarella and then the remaining patties. Pinch edges to seal. Pan fry, broil or grill to your liking. Serve with ¼ cup of Italian sauce on each burger.

LAMBBURGER

1 pound ground lamb
1 teaspoon Spike seasoning
1 tablespoon water
2 teaspoons lemon juice
Pepper to taste
1 small garlic clove
Parsley

Have butcher grind lamb shoulder, trimming away some of the fat. Mix lamb and next 4 ingredients. Crush garlic and add to lamb mix. Make 4 patties about ½ inch thick. Heat skillet and sprinkle a little Spike into skillet. Brown patties, turning often to prevent sticking. Cover and reduce heat, cook 5 to 10 minutes longer, turning occasionally. Remove to serving plate. Drain off all fat in skillet. Add ½ cup hot water and scrape loose the brown residue. Bring to boil and pour over patties. Garnish with snipped parsley.

CANDY'S BEEF PATTIES

1 pound lean ground beef
4 slices skim American cheese
1 - 4 oz. can tomato sauce
1 - 4 oz. can mushrooms, drained
Garlic powder
Pepper

Make 4 patties from the beef. Fry in a teflon skillet to your liking. Drain off excess grease. Sprinkle with garlic powder and pepper to taste. Top each patty with a slice of cheese and a mound of mushrooms. Pour tomato sauce over all, and cover for 5 to 10 minutes. Serve.

VEALBURGER

1¼ pound ground veal
1 teaspoon Spike seasoning
Pepper, to taste
1 tablespoon minced onion
1 egg, beaten
2 tablespoons oil
1 chicken bouillon cube
1 cup water

Mix veal, seasonings, onion and egg. Shape into 5 patties. Brown slowly in hot oil in heavy skillet. Drain off any excess fat. Dissolve bouillon in 1 cup of hot water, add to skillet. Cover and simmer for 45 minutes or until well done.

MEXIBURGERS

Lean ground beef
¾ cup fresh peeled green chilies, or canned and chopped
2 green onions, chopped
3 tablespoons black olives, sliced
3 tablespoons longhorn cheese, grated
Spike and pepper to taste

Make 6 thin patties with beef. Sprinkle with Spike and pepper. Mix remaining ingredients and spoon equally onto 3 patties. Top with remaining 3 patties and pinch edges to seal. Pan fry broil or grill to your liking.

ONIONBURGERS

Lean ground beef
1 large onion (any kind)
½ teaspoon Spike seasoning
Pepper to taste

Make 6 thin patties. Sprinkle with Spike and pepper. Slice onion ¼ inch thick and place 1 onion slice on each of the 3 patties. Top with the remaining patties; pinch to seal edges. Pan fry, broil or grill to your liking.

SOYBURGER

Lean ground beef
1 cup bean sprouts, fresh
½ cup green pepper diced
3 large mushrooms, sliced
2 green onions, chopped
1 tablespoon butter
Pepper to taste
½ teaspoon Spike seasoning
Soy sauce

Make 6 thin patties. Sprinkle with Spike and pepper. Saute bean sprouts, green peppers, mushrooms and onion in butter. Spoon vegetables equally on 3 patties, leaving ¼ inch clear around edge. Place remaining patties on top, encasing vegetables, and pinching to seal. Brush burgers with soy sauce; pan fry, broil or grill to your liking.

RIBS, ROASTS, STEAKS & STUFF

PRIME RIB

4 to 6 pound roast
Have butcher cut thru end bone for easy slicing, and tie roast. Place roast on wax paper, and generously coat with Italian seasoning, garlic powder pepper and Spike seasoning.
With fat side up, roast resting on the ribs, make a slit through top to the center of the roast. Insert meat thermometer. Place roast in shallow roasting pan resting on ribs.
Roast in 350 degree oven until internal temperature registers 150 degrees — or follow roasting chart to your own taste.

If you like it rare, cook at 140 degress for 90 to 105 minutes; for medium cook at 160 degrees for 105 minutes to 2 hours; for well done cook at 170 degrees for 2 hours or longer.

To slice meat, remove tie-string and bone. Slice 1 inch thick serving pieces. To make broth, remove all fat from the pan and place pan on stove burners. Add 1 to 1½ cups of hot water and soak pan for a few minutes. Turn stove burners to medium heat and stir constantly until broth boils. Pour over servings and serve.

LEMON POT ROAST
3 pound beef pot roast
2 tablespoons bacon fat
Sauce ingredients: ½ cup fresh lemon juice; ½ clove garlic; 2 tablespoons onion, minced; ½ teaspoon Spike seasoning; ½ teaspoon pepper; 1 tablespoon celery tops, minced; dash of thyme; lemon slices (optional)

Combine sauce ingredients, cover and let stand overnight. Brown pot roast in bacon fat; add sauce. Cover and simmer 2½ to 3 hours until tender. Add water during cooking if needed.

STUFFED STEAK
Pound flank steak, tenderized by butcher
3 slices of bacon, cooked until almost crisp
½ cup fresh sliced mushrooms or canned mushrooms, drained
1/3 cup grated Parmesan cheese
2 tablespoons diced onion
Garlic powder and pepper
1/3 cup Campbells Golden Mushroom Soup
1/3 cup water

Lay out steak flat on wax paper; sprinkle with garlic powder and pepper to taste. Arrange 3 slices of bacon side-by-side on steak, staying 1 inch inside the edge. Cover bacon with layer of mushrooms Sprinkle on onion and Parmesan cheese.
Starting at narrow end of the steak, roll it up in the shape of a log, tucking in the ends as you go. Tie securely. Brown steak roll in ¼ cup hot oil; drain on paper towel.
Place steak seam down in loaf pan. Mix 1/3 cup soup and 1/3 cup water. Pour over steak. Cover with foil and bake in 375 degree oven for 75 minutes.
Cool steak on cutting board for about 10 minutes; remove string and cut in 1 inch slices.

RIBBON MEATLOAF
Basic Meat Mixture:
1½ pound ground chuck or ground round
1 egg, slightly beaten
¼ cup tomato sauce
½ cup grated Parmesan cheese
1 teaspoon Italian seasoning
Pepper
1 tablespoon minced onion (optional)
Mushroom Filling:
½ cup fresh sliced mushrooms, or ½ cup canned mushrooms, drained
1 cup shredded longhorn cheese
Pepper

Mix the first 8 ingredients in the meat mixture; divide mixture into half.
Spray loaf-pan with non-stick spray. Spread half the meat mixture in bottom of loaf pan; pat lightly.
Spread on the mushroom filling. Top with the second half of the meat mixture; pat lightly. Bake in 375 degree oven for 45 minutes.
Remove from oven; drain off excess grease.
Sprinkle 2 tablespoons grated longhorn cheese on top and return to oven. Bake 5 minutes or until cheese melts. Remove from oven; slice and serve.

RIBBON MEATLOAF FILLING VARIATIONS
Cheese Filling: 1 cup shredded cheese of your choice (longhorn, Swiss, sharp cheddar, Monterey Jack, or Mozarella); 1 egg white, slightly beaten; pepper. Mix cheese and egg white and add pepper.

Egg Filling: 1 cup shredded cheese of your choice; 2 hard-boiled eggs, chopped.

Bacon Filling: 1 cup shredded cheese of your choice; 3 to 4 pieces crisp bacon, crumbled.

Sour Cream Filling: ¾ cup sour cream; 1 egg; 3 tablespoons chopped green onion. Beat egg and sour cream together, add onions.

Garden Fresh Filling: ½ cup diced celery; ½ cup shredded cheese of your choice; pepper.

Cottage Cheese Filling: ¾ cup low fat cottage cheese; ¼ cup shredded cheese of your choice; ¼ cup diced green pepper; pepper.

MEATBALLS
1 lb. lean ground beef
1 egg, beaten
1 tablespoon minced onion
Garlic powder and pepper to taste
1/4 to 1/3 cup grated Parmesan cheese

Mix all ingredients thoroughly and shape meat mixture into meatballs, whatever size you prefer. Brown meatballs in 2 tablespoons oil in a Teflon skillet. Drain on paper towel.

NOTE: I like to freeze these meatballs in quantities of six. This makes a simple, quick meal for Pat during hectic training months, when I'm kept busy preparing 6 meals a day. When I need such a quick meal, I place the frozen meatballs in foil with 1 tablespoon water and any raw vegetable such as whole mushrooms, celery, onion, tomatoes, cabbage, zucchini, etc.
Seal the foil and bake at 300 degrees for 30 to 40 minutes.
I also use these meatballs in Spicy Meatball Soup, pg.00

MARINATED LONDON BROIL
Flank steak
½ cup salad oil or low calorie Italian dressing
2 - 3 tablespoons worcestershire sauce
1 tablespoon dried minced garlic
Course-grind black pepper

Mix all ingredients and pour over steak. Cover container for 2 to 4 hours, turning occasionally. Broil or grill on barbecue to your liking. Slice at an angle in very thin slices.

LIVER AND ONIONS
1½ pounds beef liver
2 tablespoons bacon fat
1 pound onions
½ teaspoon Spike seasoning

Remove skin and tubes from liver. Brown liver on both sides in hot bacon fat over medium heat. Layer liver on one side of pan and add sliced onions. Sprinkle with Spike. Cover and cook until well-done or about 8 to 10 minutes. Serve immediately.

BROILED LIVER
1½ pounds beef liver, sliced 1 inch thick
3 tablespoons butter
1 teaspoon Spike seasoning
Pepper to taste
1 teaspoon chopped chives

Slice liver in uniform 1 inch slices, removing any skin and tubes. Brush liver on both sides with melted butter. Broil 6 minutes on each side, about 3 inches from heat. Remove to serving dish, brush with more melted butter and sprinkle with chives. Serve immediately.

Despite our persistant efforts, Pat has never developed a taste for liver, and refuses to eat it. For those who like this wonder food, these are excellent recipes.

VEAL AND LEMON
Place 8 slices of veal between 2 sheets of wax paper and pound with a meat pounder until very thin. Place veal slices on platter in single layer and cover with lemon juice. Cover and let stand for 20 to 30 minutes. Saute in 2 tablespoons of butter 3 to 4 minutes on each side, seasoning with Spike and pepper. Add ¼ cup finely chopped parsley and toss. Serve.

VEAL AND SOUR CREAM
4 veal steaks, ½ inch thick
1 clove garlic
2 tablespoons butter
¼ cup water
1 cup sour cream
1 teaspoon paprika
1 teaspoon Spike seasoning

Saute veal and garlic in butter until brown. Remove garlic. Add water, cover and simmer until tender — about 90 minutes. Add sour cream, paprika and Spike and bring to a boil. Serve immediately.

TURKEY OSCAR
3 slices of cooked turkey breast, 1 inch thick
3 slices Swiss cheese
9 Stalks of asparagus; pre-cooked or partially steamed

Place 3 asparagus stalks side-by-side on each turkey slice. Sprinkle with Spike seasoning and top with a slice of Swiss cheese. Broil until cheese melts and turkey is warmed. Serve immediately.

TROPICAL CHICKEN

2 large chicken breasts, cut into halves, deboned and skinned
4 slices canned pineapple (reserve juice)

Saute chicken breasts in butter until lightly browned. Cover and cook for 25 minutes, or until tender, turning occasionally. Place breasts in shallow baking dish and top each with a slice of pineapple. Add reserved juice to chicken bouillon to equal 1 cup of liquid and pour over chicken. Broil until pineapple turns golden brown. Serve immediately.

CHICKEN AND MUSHROOMS

4 large chicken breasts, deboned and skinned
1 pound fresh mushrooms, chopped
1 tablespoon minced onions
1/3 cup grated Parmesan cheese
Few parsley sprigs, chopped
Spike seasoning

Saute chicken breasts in butter until lightly browned. Add remaining ingredients, cover and cook, turning occasionally, for 10 to 15 minutes or until breasts are tender. Serve immediately.

PARMESAN CHICKEN

6 pieces of skinned chicken; breasts, legs or thighs
1 egg, slightly beaten
¾ cup grated Parmesan cheese

Pour cheese on piece of wax paper. Dip each piece of chicken into egg, then roll in cheese until lightly coated. Place coated chicken on cookie sheet sprayed with Mazola Non-Stick Spray. Bake in 375 degree oven for 45 minutes until golden brown. Use pancake turner to remove chicken to paper toweling to get off excess oil. Serve hot or cold.

STUFFED GAME HENS

2 frozen cornish game hens, thawed
Garlic powder and pepper

Stuffing: 1 cup mushrooms, fresh or canned; ½ cup diced celery; 2 tablespoons diced onions; 1 teaspoon Rosemary.

Rinse and drain game hens. Pepper and garlic powder inside cavity. Toss stuffing ingredients lightly and stuff each cavity. Cross the legs and tie. Place in shallow baking pan and cover with foil. Bake in 375 degree oven for 30 minutes. Uncover and bake additional 45 minutes, basting occasionally with pan drippings.

TARRAGON CHICKEN IN WINE

6 chicken breasts, skinned and boned
1 cup dry white wine
½ cup fresh chopped parsley
1 tablespoon flour
2 tablespoons tarragon
Garlic powder and pepper
2 tablespoons margarine

Place chicken breasts on wax paper. Sprinkle with flour, tarragon, garlic powder and pepper. Cover with a second sheet of wax paper and flatten with a meat mallet.

Melt margarine over medium high heat in a large teflon skillet, and add chicken, cooking 5 minutes on each side. Place cooked chicken on serving plate. Add wine to skillet and boil for 1 minute, stirring constantly. Remove from heat and add fresh parsley. Pour wine mixture over chicken and serve.

BAKED ITALIAN CHICKEN

6 to 8 pieces skinned chicken, legs, thighs or breasts
1 cup diced fresh tomatoes
Italian seasoning
Garlic powder and pepper

Coat 2 inch deep baking pan with Mazola Non-Stick Spray. Put 2 tablespoons Italian seasoning and garlic powder and pepper to taste in a plastic bag. Toss 2 pieces of chicken at a time, coating generously. Arrange chicken on baking pan and cover with foil. Bake in 375 degree oven for 30 minutes. Remove foil and sprinkle with diced tomatoes. Return uncovered to oven and bake 30 more minutes.

GRILLED FISH

2 - 3 pounds of fresh fish; your choice
Pepper and Spike
Garlic powder
1/3 cup of beer

Use a hamburger rack for barbecuing (cake racks may also be used). Spray racks generously with non-stick spray and arrange fish on racks in single layer. Place rack on grill over hot coals. Baste generously with beer, pepper and garlic powder mix. Cook 5 to 7 minutes on each side or until center of fish will flake when poked with fork.

SALMON STEAKS

Marinade sauce ingredients: ½ cup unsaturated oil; ¼ cup snipped parsley; ¼ cup lemon juice; 2 tablespoons grated onion; ½ teaspoon dry mustard; ½ teaspoon Spike seasoning; dash of pepper.

Marinade 4 fresh or frozen (thawed) salmon steaks in shallow baking dish at room temperature for about 2 hours, turning occasionally. Drain off sauce and reserve for basting.
Brown steaks lightly in 2 tablespoons of margarine, then bake in 350 degree oven for 30 minutes, basting occasionally with sauce.

BROILED LOBSTER

Place thawed rock lobster tails on broiler pan and brush with melted butter. Broil under medium heat, brushing occasionally with butter for 5 minutes. Sprinkle with grated Parmesan cheese and continue broiling for 3 to 5 minutes until cheese is golden brown.

SHRIMP DELIGHT

2½ pounds of fresh shrimp, large size
1½ quarts of water
½ cup chopped celery tops
1 can of beer

Bring water, celery tops and beer mix to a hard boil in large kettle. Add shrimp and continue to boil 3 to 5 minutes until shrimp shells turn bright pink. Strain off water. Remove outer shells from shrimp, clean and de-vein. Arrange shrimp on platter and sprinkle with fresh lemon juice. Serve warm or cold.

COD AND CHEESE SAUCE

1½ pounds of fresh or frozen cod fillets
½ cup mayonnaise (imitation-zero carbohydrates)
Dash of cayenne
1 tablespoon chopped capers
1 tablespoon chopped chives
Few sprigs of parsley, chopped
½ cup grated sharp cheddar cheese
1 egg white

Place fish on greased broiler rack. Broil under medium heat for 8 to 14 minutes. Sprinkle with salt and pepper. Combine mayonnaise, cayenne, capers, chives, parsley and cheese. Beat egg white until stiff, and fold into dressing; Spread on fish and broil for 5 minutes until sauce is puffed.

BAKED FISH, PIQUANT

1½ pounds fresh or frozen cod, flounder, sole, haddock or halibut.
1 teaspoon grated onion
1 teaspoon Spike seasoning
1/8 teaspoon white pepper
¼ cup melted butter
Juice of 1 lemon
Paprika
Minced parsley

Cut fish in serving pieces and arrange in greased shallow baking dish. Sprinkle with Spike and pepper. Combine lemon, butter and onion, and pour over fish. Sprinkle with paprika. Bake in preheated oven at 325 degrees for 30 minutes. Sprinkle with parsley.

BAKED FISH

2 pounds fish, fresh or frozen
Pepper and Spike
Garlic powder
Lemon juice
1 tablespoon parsley
1 tablespoon butter

Melt butter and add pepper, lemon juice and parsley. Brush fish with butter and bake covered for 30 minutes in 350 degree oven. Serve.

FISH WITH WINE AND TOMATOES

2 pounds white fish fillets, fresh or frozen
1 medium onion, finely chopped
Chopped parsley
1 garlic clove, minced
1 tablespoon salad oil
2 tablespoons butter
1 cup white wine
2 peeled tomatoes, chopped
2 tablespoons tomato juice
Juice of 1 lemon

Place in a baking dish half the oil and some of the onion and parsley. Place fish on top, then pour over it the rest of the oil, lemon juice, tomato juice, garlic, wine and tomatoes. Pepper lightly. Cover and bake in 350 degree oven for 30 minutes.

LAMB STEAKS IN MARINADE

2 pounds lamb sliced from leg, 1 inch thick
3 tablespoons each of olive oil and vinegar
½ teaspoon salt
1 onion, minced
Few sprigs of parsley, chopped
Few rosemary leaves, chopped
Butter

Pound meat 3/4 inch in thickness. Put in bowl. Mix remaining ingredients except butter, and pour over meat. Refrigerate several hours or overnight. Saute meat quickly on both sides in small amount of hot butter in skillet. Heat marinade and pour over meat on serving platter.

GARLIC LAMB STEAKS

Crush 1 garlic clove and let test in ½ cup of olive oil. Broil lamb steaks over brisk fire from 3 to 6 minutes on each side, brushing them with garlic oil. Season to taste.

ZIPPY LAMB SHANKS

4 lamb shanks
Pepper
2 tablespoons oil
1 medium onion, sliced
½ cup sliced celery
1 garlic clove, minced
½ cup catsup
1½ teaspoon worcestershire sauce

Season lamb shanks with pepper. In skillet, brown meat in hot oil. Combine onion, celery, garlic, catsup, ½ cup water and worcestershire sauce. Add meat. Simmer covered for 1½ hours or until meat is tender. Skim off excess fat and serve.

CURRIED LAMB CHOPS

6 lamb chops
1 tablespoon oil
1 cup fresh peaches or unsweetened
    canned peaches
1 tablespoon lemon juice
¼ cup sliced green onion with tops
½ teaspoon curry powder
½ cup water

Brown chops in hot oil, season with pepper. Drain off excess fat. Add remaining ingredients; cover and simmer about 1 hour.

BASIC LAMB CHOPS

4 to 6 lamb chops
Pepper and Spike
Minced onion
½ cup fresh or canned mushrooms

Brown lamb chops in teflon skillet coated with non-stick spray. Pepper. Add onion and mushrooms, and cover. Continue cooking on low heat for 45 minutes, turning occasionally.

A DESSERT IS A DESSERT IS A DESSERT

A dessert is a dessert no matter how you slice it. So while training, Pat usually limits himself to fresh low carbohydrate fruit for his sweet tooth. And living in Phoenix, Arizona where our summer temperatures average 105 degrees (in the shade!), he craves anything cold or frozen. My desserts are therefore a combination of both cold and frozen fruit dishes.

FLUFFY PARFAITS
1 package unsweetened gelatin, any flavor
2 egg whites
3 teaspoons fructose

Prepare gelatin following package directions, omitting sugar. Chill until lightly thickened. Beat egg whites, adding a little fructose at a time until stiff. Fold or beat into gelatin. Spoon into 4 parfait glasses. Chill and serve.

SNOW-CAPPED PEACHES
3 medium-size fresh peaches, or unsweetened canned peach-halves
2 egg whites
1½ teaspoon fructose
1/8 teaspoon cream of tartar
Cinnamon
Diced walnuts

Carefully peel fresh peaches, cut in half and remove seeds. Place halved peaches in pie-plate, cup side up. Sprinkle with cinnamon and walnuts. Beat egg whites, cream of tartar and fructose until stiff. Spoon a mound of egg whites on each peach cup. Bake in preheated oven at 450 degrees until golden brown (3 to 5 minutes). Serve warm or cold.

FROZEN FRUIT BITES
Dip small clusters of seedless green grapes in prepared meringue, sweetened with fructose. Place on cookie sheet and freeze. Also good with strawberries.

CANTALOUPE ICE
Dice 1 fresh cantaloupe and combine in a blender with 1/2 to 3/4 cup water. When thoroughly blended, fill popsicle maker or paper cups and freeze.

FROZEN PEACH WHIP
1 cup water
½ cup skim milk
1 teaspoon vanilla
2 tablespoons yogurt
3 peaches scrubbed, cut and seeds removed
1 teaspoon fructose

Whip all ingredients in blender and freeze in paper cups. Also excellent with other low carbohydrate fruits, such as strawberries and canteloupe.

MERINGUE FRUIT PIE
3 egg whites, at room temperature
1/8 teaspoon cream of tartar
Dash of salt
¼ cup fructose

Beat egg whites until foamy; add cream of tartar and salt. Gradually beat in fructose. Continue beating until stiff, glossy peaks form. With the back of a spoon spread meringue in 9 inch pie-plate sprayed with non-stick coating; cover bottom and form sides ½ inch higher than plate rim. Bake in preheated 250 degree oven for 1 hour or until firm to touch. Turn oven off. Leave in closed oven to dry until oven is cool. Fill with desired low carbohydrate fruits such as strawberries or peaches. Serve immediately as crust will soon dissolve.

FRIED APPLES
In a small sauce pan melt 1 tablespoon butter. Slice 2 medium apples unpeeled, and gently saute. Sprinkle with 1 teaspoon fructose and some cinnamon to taste (optional). Cover and simmer to desired tenderness. Sprinkle with walnut bits and serve warm.

SPICY PEACH CUPS

1 package Jell-O unsweetened gelatin dessert (any flavor)
5 teaspoons fructose or 3 tablepoons raw honey
¼ teaspoon cinnamon
1 cup boiling water
1 cup cold water
1½ cups fresh peaches, diced

Dissolve gelatin and cinnamon in boiling water. Stir in cold water and chill until slightly thickened. Fold in peaches and spoon into individual dessert dishes. Chill until firm
Serve with D-Zerta Whipped Topping, if desired.

BAKED EGG CUSTARD

2 cups skim milk
¼ cup plus 1 teaspoon fructose
1/8 teaspoon salt
3 eggs, beaten
½ teaspoon vanilla
Nutmeg

In a saucepan combine milk and fructose. Heat over medium heat without stirring, until a thick layer begins to form on top. Remove from heat and add eggs, vanilla and salt. Beat well. Pour into 4 oven-safe custard cups sprayed with non-stick coating. Place cups in a pan of water so water is about half way up on cups. Sprinkle nutmeg on top of each custard cup.
Bake in preheated oven at 325 degrees for 45 to 50 minutes. Remove cups from pan of water. Serve warm or cold.

BAKED APPLES

4 Rome Beauty cooking apples
¼ teaspoon cinnamon
1 cup Rocotta cheese
Nutmeg
1 cup water
1 tablespoon honey (optional)

Core apples and peel about one-third way down from stem end. Sprinkle cinnamon inside each apple. Arrange in shallow baking dish and bake at 350 degrees for 40 to 45 minutes. Mix Ricotta and nutmeg to taste. Spoon cheese into cooked apple cavity and continue baking 15 minutes. Brush with honey the last 5 minutes. Serve warm or cold.

BEVERAGES

Pat isn't much on fancy beverages, but over the years he has found a few that he enjoys drinking (during competitive training he mostly drinks water).

PERRIER WATER

With a twist of lime, this is Pat's favorite drink.

LEMON WATER

Add fresh or concentrated lemon juice to water. Sugar substitutes to taste.

ICED COFFEE

8 oz. decaffeinated coffee with 1 teaspoon of powdered skim milk and a pinch of cinnamon, on the rocks.

SPICED TEA

4 cups boiling water
4 teaspoons loose tea
6 whole cloves broken into pieces
½ teaspoon dried orange peel
1/8 teaspoon cinnamon

Pour boiling water on all ingredients in heat-proof container. Cover, steep for 3 to 5 minutes. Stir and strain. Serve hot or cold.

With little ones in the house I make gallons of Kool-Aid every day. For two years Pat drank unsweetened Kool-Aid because it was always on-hand, eventually developing a taste for it. He won the Mr. USA title during this period, and acquired the reputation of having trained for the contest on Kool-Aid. Try it, you might like it.

IX
ATHLETE'S VITAMIN and MINERAL GUIDE

When it comes to vitamin and mineral supplements, there are many different opinions about how much to take and how useful they are. Personally, I feel they are beneficial if taken properly and with some degree of knowledge.

Each individual's metabolism is unique and each supplement program will vary to some extent. It is an individual decision as to what nutritional supplemental program suits you best. That's why I strongly recommend potential bodybuilders to research vitamins and minerals for themselves and, if possible, seek advice from a nutritionist or biochemist in setting up their personal supplement program.

Generally speaking, there are a few basic principles that can apply to almost everyone supplementing his or her own diet.

Fat-soluble vitamins are best absorbed if taken with meals and are stored in the body, primarily in the liver. Water-soluable vitamins are quickly removed from the body by the kidneys and therefore generally taken two to four times a day. All vitamins complement each other and likewise, many minerals seem to be co-workers with each other and particular vitamins. That's why individual research on vitamins and minerals is so important to a personal supplement program. A lot of benefit can be wasted by not understanding the whole picture on vitamins and minerals.

The following is a basic chart on vitamins and minerals, their benefits, and the foods they are found in naturally.

VITAMIN GUIDE

VITAMIN	BENEFITS	NATURAL SOURCES
Vitamin A RETINOL (Fat-Soluble)	Eyes, skin and hair. Helps in maintaining healthy mucous membranes in the body.	Carrots, lettuce, tomatoes, sweet potatoes, peas, liver, eggs and dairy foods.
Vitamin B_1 THIAMINE (Water Soluble)	The nervous system and circulation. Aids digestion and the metabolism of protein and carbohydrates.	Brewer's Yeast, wheat germ, whole grain cereals, nuts, soy beans, milk products, eggs, meat, fish, and leafy green vegetables.
Vitamin B_2 RIBOFLAVIN (Water-Soluble)	Essential for growth and general health.	Milk, cheese, fish, liver, poultry, eggs, whole grain bread, and cereals.
Vitamin B_3 NIACIN or NIACINAMIDE (Water-Soluble)	Aids in protein and carbohydrate metabolism.	Meat, liver, fish, nuts, butter, poultry, eggs, whole grain bread and cereal.

VITAMIN GUIDE (continued)

VITAMIN	BENEFITS	NATURAL SOURCES
Vitamin B$_5$ PANTOTHENIC ACID (Water-Soluble)	Involved in adrenal gland function. Required to fight stress.	Whole grain cereals, animal tissues.
Vitamin B$_6$ PYRIDOXINE (Water-Soluble)	Protein, fat, and sugar metabolism and the central nervous system.	Corn, lima beans, liver and ham.
Vitamin B$_{12}$ CYANOBOBALAMIN (Water-Soluble)	Involved in the production of red blood cells.	Milk, eggs, liver, Brewer's Yeast, sunflower seeds, bananas, and raw wheat germ.

OTHER IMPORTANT MEMBERS OF B-COMPLEX

VITAMIN	BENEFITS	NATURAL SOURCES
Biotin	Involved in metabolism of fats, carbohydrates, and proteins. Related to hair growth and maintenance.	Brewer's Yeast, eggs, soy beans, liver and kidneys.
Inositol	May be involved in hair growth and healthy heart muscles. There is evidence it may reduce blood cholesterol.	Fruits, whole grains, Brewer's Yeast, wheat germ, and organ meats.
Folic Acid	Co-worker with Vitamin B$_{12}$ and is involved in the formation of red blood cells.	Green leafy vegetables, Brewer's Yeast, wheat germ, eggs, milk, eggs, and yogurt.
Choline	Essential for fat metabolism.	Eggs, liver, Brewer's Yeast, wheat germ, and green leafy vegetables.

VITAMIN	BENEFITS	NATURAL SOURCES
Vitamin C ASCORBIC ACID (Water-Soluble)	Detoxifies many poisonous substances in the body and is important in the healing process. Aids in red blood cell formation and helps fight stress.	Citrus fruits, strawberries, potatoes, green bell peppers and raw greens.
Vitamin D CALCIFEROL (Fat-Soluble)	Important in infancy and adolescence for healthy teeth and bones. Required throughout life for proper calcium metabolism.	Fish, liver, oils, egg yolks, milk, sunflower seeds, and mushrooms.
Vitamin E TOCOPHEROL	Vital to normal reproduction. Research shows evidence that Vitamin E may slow the aging process and prevent heart disease.	Whole grains, wheat germ, nuts, sprouts, eggs, and green leafy vegetables.

MINERAL GUIDE

MINERAL	BENEFITS	NATURAL SOURCES
CALCIUM (a co-worker with) (phosphorous)	Necessary for normal growth and building bones and teeth. Balances potassium and sodium for muscle tone, regulates heartbeat and assists in blood clotting.	Milk, and cheese, sesame seeds, and dark leafy green vegetables.
CHLORINE	Due to the consumption of chlorinated water, chlorine is rarely deficient. Its primary function is in the production of hydochloric acid in the stomach.	Avocados, tomatoes, cabbage, kale, celery, cucumber, pineapple, salt water. fish and kelp.
COBALT	An integral part of Vitamin B_{12}. Involved in the uptake of oxygen by cells in their life process.	Liver, leafy green vegetables.
COPPER	Essential to iron absorption. Involved in protein metabolism and assists the body to oxidize Vitamin C.	Green leafy vegetables, whole grains, almonds, beans, peas, prunes, raisins and liver.
FLUORINE	Essential to bone and tooth building. In excess, sodium fluorine, the chemical waste product, can cause mottled teeth and toxicity.	Sea water, naturally hard water. Sunflower seeds, milk, cheese, garlic, carrots and green leafy vegetables.
IODINE	Essential for the health of the thyroid gland. Helps to regulate many metabolic functions in the body.	Kelp, turnip greens, garlic, pears, pineapple, artichokes, citrus fruits, egg yolks, seafood, fish, liver, oil.
IRON	Vital for the formation of hemoglobin which carries oxygen to every cell of the body.	Black molasses, prunes, raisins, Brewer's Yeast, whole grain cereals, apricots, bananas, spinach, beets, sunflower seeds, walnuts, liver and egg yolks.
MAGNESIUM	Catalyst in many enzyme sytems. Needed for normal contraction of muscles. Necessary for efficient synthesis of certain amino acids. It is a natural tranquilizer.	Green leafy vegetables, brussel sprouts, spinach, blueberries, grapefruit, oranges, bran, peas, and wheat germ.

MINERAL GUIDE (continued)

MINERAL	BENEFITS	NATURAL SOURCES
MOLYBDENUM	A component of certain enzymes, and very rarely deficient. It is involved in mobilizing iron from the liver's reserves.	Whole cereals, Brewer's Yeast, dark green vegetables.
PHOSPHORUS	Needed for building bones and teeth. It is an important factor in fat and carbohydrate metabolism. Needed for healthy nerves.	Whole grains, nuts, seeds, egg yolks, dairy products and dried fruits.
POTASSIUM	Important for proper muscle contraction and heart function. Helps stimulate kidneys and acts with sodium to regulate fluids. It is necessary for normal health of adrenals and assists in the conversion of glucose to glycogen.	All vegetables, oranges, bananas, milk, sunflower seeds, nuts, whole grains.
SELENIUM	Anti-oxidant; closely related to Vitamin E.	Brewer's Yeast, seafood, milk, eggs and most vegetables.
SULFUR	Involved in the maintenance of healthy skin, hair and finger nails. Abundantly bound to protein intake, thus rarely deficient.	Onions, celery, string beans, soy beans, meat and fish.
SODIUM	Associated with potassium and chlorine, sodium regulates the body fluids and internal fluid PH.	Celery, romaine lettuce, watermelon, kelp and sea salt.
ZINC	The second largest quantity trace mineral in the body. (Iron is the first.) Necessary for absorption and activity of vitamins, particularly the B-complex. Increases healing of burns and other wounds. Essential for normal function of the prostate gland.	Wheat germ, sunflower seeds, Brewer's Yeast, milk, eggs, green leafy vegetables, onions and oysters.

X

A FOOD GUIDE FOR BODYBUILDING

FOOD DESCRIPTION	UNIT OF MEASURE	PRO-TEIN Gm.	FAT Gm.	CARBO-HYDRATES Gm.	CAL-ORIES (energy)
Almonds, dried, un-blanched, shelled	1 cup	26.4	76.8	27.8	848
Almonds, in shell as purchased	1 cup	7.4	21.6	7.8	238
Apples, raw as purchased	3" dia.	.6	.8	30.1	117
Apples, cubed or sliced	1 cup	.4	.6	21.2	83
Apples, dried and uncooked	1 cup	1.6	1.1	83.4	315
Apple Butter	1 cup	1.1	2.3	128.0	518
Apple Butter	1 Tbsp.	.1	.1	8.2	33
Apple Juice, fresh or canned	1 cup	.2	(0)	34.4	124
Applesauce, canned (unsweetened)	1 cup	.5	.5	26.1	100
Applesauce, canned (sweetened)	1 cup	.5	.3	50.0	184
Apricots, raw as purchased	3 pcs.	1.1	.1	13.8	54

FOOD DESCRIPTION	UNIT OF MEASURE	PRO-TEIN Gm.	FAT Gm.	CARBO-HYDRATES Gm.	CAL-ORIES (energy)
Apricots, canned halves in water	1 cup	1.2	.2	19.8	77
Apricots, canned havles in syrup	1 cup	1.5	.3	54.8	205
Apricots, dried, sulphured, uncooked	1 cup	7.8	.6	100.4	393
Asparagus, cooked, cut in spears	1 cup	4.2	.4	6.3	36
Asparagus, canned, green with liquid	6 sprs	2.4	.4	3.7	22
Avocados, cubed 1/2" squares	1 cup	2.6	40.1	7.8	372
Avocados, (3½" x 3¼" half)	1/2 pc.	1.9	30.1	5.8	279
Bacon, med. fat, broiled or fried	2 slcs.	4.0	8.0	.2	97
Bacon, Canadian, as purchased	4 oz.	25.1	17.0	.3	262
Bananas, raw, as purchased 6" x 1½"	1 med.	1.2	.2	23.0	88
Barley, pearled, light, dry	1 cup	16.6	2.0	160.0	708
Beans, red kidney, canned or cooked	1 cup	14.6	1.0	42.0	230
Beans, other common, raw	1 cup	40.7	3.0	117.0	642
Beans, other common, canned & baked	1 cup	15.1	7.8	50.1	325
Beans, lima, raw and cooked	1 lb.	22.7	1.8	83.1	432

FOOD DESCRIPTION	UNIT MEASURE	PROTEIN Gm.	FAT Gm.	CARBO-HYDRATES Gm.	CALORIES (energy)
Beans, lima, raw and cooked	1 cup	8.0	.6	29.3	152
Beans, lima, canned no liquid	1 cup	8.0	.6	29.3	152
Beans, snap, green, cooked	1 cup	1.8	.2	5.9	27
Beans, snap, green, canned	1 cup	1.8	.2	5.9	27
Beans, wax or yellow, canned with liquid	1 cup	2.4	.2	10.0	43
Beans, wax or yellow, canned, drained	1 cup	1.8	.2	5.9	27
Beans, soya, whole, mature, dried	1 cup	73.3	38.3	73.1	695
Beans, soya, sprouts, raw	1 cup	6.6	1.5	5.7	49
Bean soup, condensed	11 oz.	21.5	12.8	73.6	481
Bean soup, ready to serve	1 cup	8.5	5.0	29.5	191
Beef chuck, cooked, with bone	1 lb.	96.0	81.0	(0)	1,140
Beef, chuck, cooked without bone	1 lb.	118.0	100.0	(0)	1,406
Beef, chuck, cooked, without bone	3 oz.	22.0	19.0	(0)	265
Beef, flank, cooked, with bone	1 lb.	110.0	101.0	(0)	1,381
Beef, flank, cooked, without bone	1 lb.	114.0	104.0	(0)	1,425

FOOD DESCRIPTION	UNIT MEASURE	PROTEIN Gm.	FAT Gm.	CARBOHYDRATES Gm.	CALORIES (energy)
Beef flank, cooked, without bone	3 oz.	21.0	20.0	(0)	270
Beef hamburger, (regular as purchased)	1 lb.	100.0	136.0	(0)	1,654
Beef hamburger, (regular as purchased	3 oz.	19.0	26.0	(0)	316
Beef, hamburger, lean (ground round steak)	1 lb.	123.0	59.0	(0)	1,057
Beef, hamburger, lean (ground round steak)	3 oz.	23.0	11.0	(0)	197
Beef, porterhouse, with bone	1 lb.	86.0	100.0	(0)	1,269
Beef, porterhouse, without bone	1 lb.	104.0	123.0	(0)	1,554
Beef, porterhouse, without bone	3 oz.	20.0	23.0	(0)	293
Beef, rib roast, with bone	1 lb.	79.0	79.0	(0)	1,050
Beef, rib roast, without bone	1 lb.	109.0	109.0	(0)	1,449
Beef, rib roast, without bone	3 oz.	20.0	20.0	(0)	266
Beef, round, with bone	1 lb.	107.0	51.0	(0)	917
Beef, round, without bone	1 lb.	123.0	59.0	(0)	1,057
Beef, round, without bone	3 oz.	23.0	11.0	(0)	197
Beef, rump, with bone	1 lb.	65.0	99.0	(0)	1,171
Beef, rump, without bone	1 lb.	95.0	145.0	(0)	1,714

FOOD DESCRIPTION	UNIT MEASURE	PROTEIN Gm.	FAT Gm.	CARBOHYDRATES Gm.	CALORIES (energy)
Beef, rump, without bone	3 oz.	18.0	27.0	(0)	320
Beef, sirloin, with bone	1 lb.	91.0	87.0	(0)	1,173
Beef, sirloin, without bone	1 lb.	104.0	100.0	(0)	1,346
Beef, sirloin, without bone	3 oz.	20.0	19.0	(0)	257
Beef, canned corned beef hash	3 oz.	11.7	5.2	6.1	120
Beef, canned roast beef	3 oz.	21.0	11.0	(0)	189
Beef, canned, strained infant food	1 oz.	4.9	1.0	(0)	221
Beef, canned corned beef, lean	3 oz.	22.5	7.0	(0)	159
Beef, canned corned beef, medium fat	3 oz.	21.5	10.0	(0)	182
Beef, canned corned beef, fat	3 oz.	20.0	15.0	(0)	221
Beef, dried and chipped	1 cup	56.6	10.4	(0)	336
Beef, dried and chipped	2 oz.	19.4	3.6	(0)	115
Beef & Vegetable Stew (average recipe)	1 cup	12.9	19.3	16.7	252
Beef Soup, condensed	11 oz.	15.0	8.4	27.8	481
Beef Soup, ready to serve	1 cup	6.0	3.5	11.0	100

FOOD DESCRIPTION	UNIT OF MEASURE	PRO-TEIN Gm.	FAT Gm.	CARBO-HYDRATES Gm.	CAL-ORIES (energy)
Beef Broth, consomme bouillon, cond.	11 oz.	6.0	(0)	(0)	26
Beef Broth, consomme bouillon, ready to serve	1 cup	2.0	(0)	(0)	9
Beer (reg. 4% alcohol)	1 cup	1.4	(0)	10.6	114
Beets, common red, fresh cooked	1 cup	1.6	.2	16.2	68
Beets, common red, canned, with liquid	1 cup	2.2	.2	19.4	82
Beets, common red, canned, drained, liquid	1 cup	1.6	.2	16.2	69
Beet Greens, common, cooked	1 cup	2.0	.4	8.1	39
Beverages, carbonated, ginger ale 8 fl. oz.	1 cup	(0)	(0)	21.0	80
Beverages, carbonated, others incl. colas	1 cup	(0)	(0)	28.0	107
Biscuits, baking powder, unenriched flour	2-1/2"	3.1	4.0	19.8	129
Biscuits, baking powder, enriched flour	2-1/2"	3.1	4.0	19.8	129
Biscuits, baking powder, enriched flour, self-rising	2-1/2"	3.0	4.1	19.0	127
Blackberries, fresh	1 cup	1.7	1.4	18.0	82
Blackberries, canned, water packed	1 cup	2.2	1.7	22.9	104
Blackberries, canned, incl. syrup pack	1 cup	1.8	.5	57.2	216
Blueberries, fresh	1 cup	.8	.8	21.1	85

FOOD DESCRIPTION	UNIT OF MEASURE	PRO-TEIN (Gm.)	FAT (Gm.)	CARBO-HYDRATES (Gm.)	CAL-ORIES (energy)
Blueberries, canned, water packed	1 cup	1.0	1.0	21.8	90
Blueberries, canned, syrup pack	1 cup	1.0	1.0	64.7	245
Blueberries, frozen, without sugar	3 oz.	.5	.5	12.8	52
Bluefish, baked (portion of 3½" x 3½")	1 pc.	34.2	5.2	(0)	193
Bluefish, fried (portion of 3½" x 3½")	1 pc.	34.0	14.7	7.0	307
Bologna, (1" x 1½" dia. portion)	1 pc.	31.2	33.5	7.6	467
Boston Brown Bread, (slice, 3" x ¼")	1 sl.	2.3	1.0	22.1	105
Bouillon cubes, (5/8" sq. cube)	1 cube	.2	.1	(0)	2
Bouillon Soup, condensed	11 oz.	6.0	(0)	(0)	26
Bouillon Soup, ready to serve	1 cup	2.0	(0)	(0)	9
Brains, all animals	3 oz.	8.8	7.3	.7	106
Bran cereal, (breakfast type) all bran	1 cup	7.2	2.0	44.5	145
Bran cereal, (breakfast type) 40% bran	1 cup	4.3	.8	31.5	117
Bran, raisin	1 cup	4.5	.9	39.3	149
Brazil nuts, shelled	1 cup	20.2	92.3	15.4	905
Brazil nuts, in shell	1 cup	8.8	40.2	6.7	394
Bread, cracked wheat (1/2" thick slice)	1 sl.	2.0	.5	11.0	60

FOOD DESCRIPTION	UNIT OF MEASURE	PROTEIN Gm.	FAT Gm.	CARBOHYDRATES Gm.	CALORIES (energy)
Bread, French style	1/4 lb.	9.2	3.3	76.5	306
Bread, Italian style	1/4 lb.	9.9	.9	60.9	374
Bread, raisin, (1/2" thick slice)	1 sl.	1.6	.7	13.3	65
Bread, rye, American (1/2" thick slice)	1 sl.	2.1	.3	12.1	57
Bread, white (1/2" thick slice)	1 sl.	2.0	.7	11.9	63
Bread, whole wheat (1/2" thick slice)	1 sl.	2.1	.6	11.3	55
Breakfast cereals, mixed	1 cup	9.0	.2	37.6	177
Broccoli, fresh, cooked, flower stalks	1 cup	5.0	.3	8.2	44
Brussel sprouts, cooked, fresh	1 cup	5.7	.6	11.6	60
Buckwheat flour, dark sifted	1 cup	11.5	2.5	70.6	340
Buckwheat flour, light sifted	1 cup	6.3	1.2	77.9	342
Butter	1 Tbsp.	.1	11.3	.1	100
Butter (pat or square)	7 gm.	(0)	5.7	(0)	50
Buttermilk	1 cup	8.5	.2	12.4	86
Cabbage, fresh cooked	1 cup	2.4	.3	9.0	40
Cantaloupes, fresh (5" diameter)	1/2 pc.	1.1	.4	8.3	35
Cantaloupes, fresh (diced)	1/2 cup	.9	.3	6.1	30

FOOD DESCRIPTION	UNIT OF MEASURE	PRO-TEIN	FAT	CARBO-HYDRATES	CAL-ORIES
		Gm.	Gm.	Gm.	(energy)
Carrots, fresh 5 ½" x 1")	1 pc.	.6	.2	4.6	21
Carrots, canned, liquid drained	1 cup	.9	.7	9.3	44
Cashew nuts, roasted or cooked	1 oz.	5.2	13.7	7.7	164
Cauliflower, fresh cooked	1 cup	2.9	.2	5.9	30
Celery, raw bleached (3 small or 1 large stalk)	50 gms.	.6	.1	1.8	9
Cereal foods, pre-cooked type	1 oz.	4.0	.7	20.8	103
Chard, fresh, cooked	1 cup	4.6	.7	8.4	47
Cheese, blue mold domestic type	1 oz.	6.1	6.6	.6	104
Cheese, Camembert	1 oz.	5.0	7.0	.5	85
Cheese, cheddar	1 oz.	7.1	9.1	.6	113
Cheese, cheddar, processed	1 oz.	6.6	8.5	.6	105
Cheese, cottage	1 cup	43.9	1.1	4.5	215
Cheese, cottage	1 oz.	5.5	.1	.6	27
Cheese, limburger	1 oz.	6.0	7.9	.6	97
Cheese, Parmesan	1 oz.	10.2	7.4	.8	112
Cheese, Swiss	1 oz.	7.8	7.9	.5	105
Cheese, Swiss processed	1 oz.	7.5	7.6	.5	101

FOOD DESCRIPTION	UNIT OF MEASURE	PROTEIN Gm.	FAT Gm.	CARBO-HYDRATES Gm.	CALORIES (energy)
Cherries, fresh, sweet or sour	1 cup	1.2	.5	15.8	65
Cherries, canned, pitted, sour or sweet	1 cup	2.0	.8	30.2	122
Chicken, broilers (1/2 average bird)	8 oz.	44.4	15.8	(0)	332
Chicken, canned and boned	3 oz.	25.3	6.8	(0)	169
Chicken, frying pieces, breast	8 oz.	47.0	1.0	(0)	210
Chicken, frying pieces, leg portions	5 oz.	29.1	3.8	(0)	159
Chicken, roasting, boned	4 Oz.	22.9	14.3	(0)	227
Chicken, stewing hens, boned	4 oz.	20.4	28.4	(0)	342
Chicken soup, condensed	11 oz.	8.4	5.9	24.6	187
Chicken soup, ready to serve	1 cup	3.5	2.5	9.5	75
Chili con carne (without bones)	1/3 cup	2.8	12.8	4.9	170
Chili sauce	1 Tbsp.	.5	.1	4.0	17
Chocolate, bitter or unsweetened	1 oz.	1.6	15.0	8.4	142
Chocolate, sweetened plain	1 oz.	.6	8.4	17.8	133
Chocolate Beverages, milk made	1 cup	8.2	12.5	26.2	239

FOOD DESCRIPTION	UNIT OF MEASURE	PRO-TEIN Gm.	FAT Gm.	CARBO-HYDRATES Gm.	CAL-ORIES (energy)
Chocolate syrup	1 Tbsp.	.2	.2	11.3	42
Clams, fresh, meat only	4 oz.	14.5	1.6	3.9	92
Clams, canned, solids & liquids	3 oz.	6.7	.9	1.8	44
Cocoa beverage, milk made	1 cup	9.5	11.5	27.2	298
Cocoanut, fresh, meat only	1/2 cup	1.5	15.6	6.3	161
Cocoanut Milk	1 cup	.7	1.0	12.0	60
Cod, fresh, cooked	4 oz.	18.7	.5	(0)	84
Cod, dried	1 oz.	23.2	.8	(0)	106
Cole slaw, fresh grated	1 cup	1.6	7.3	9.2	102
Cookies, plain assorted types (3" dia. 1/2")	25 gm.	1.5	3.2	18.8	109
Cookies, wafer type (2-1/8" dia.)	2 pc.	.6	1.3	7.5	44
Corn, sweet, yellow or white, kernels only	1 cup	4.5	1.2	33.3	140
Corn, sweet, yellow or white, fresh	1 ear	2.7	.7	20.3	84
Corn, canned, solids and liquids	1 cup	5.1	1.3	41.2	170
Cornbread or muffins (2½" dia.)	1 pc.	3.5	2.7	16.7	103

FOOD DESCRIPTION	UNIT OF MEASURE	PROTEIN Gm.	FAT Gm.	CARBOHYDRATES Gm.	CALORIES (energy)
Cornflakes, (regular breakfast type)	1 cup	2.0	.0	21.2	96
Corn Grits, cooked	1 cup	2.9	.2	26.6	122
Corn Meal, whole, ground, cooked	1 cup	2.6	.5	25.5	119
Crabs, Atlantic or Pacific hard shelled	3 oz.	14.4	2.5	1.1	89
Crackers, graham (4 small or 2 medium)	14 gm.	1.1	1.4	10.4	55
Crackers, saltines (w. crackers 2" sq.)	8 gm.	.7	.9	5.7	34
Crackers, soda, plain type (2 pcs. 2½" sq.)	11 gm.	1.1	1.1	8.0	47
Crackers, soda, oyster type (10 pcs.)	10 gm	1.0	1.0	7.3	43
Cranberries, fresh	1 cup	.5	.8	12.8	54
Cranberry sauce, sweetened, cand. or cooked	1 cup	.3	.8	142.4	549
Cream, light table or coffee	1 Tbsp.	.4	3.0	.6	30
Cream, heavy or whipping	1 Tbsp.	.3	5.2	.5	49
Cress, water, leaves & stems	1 lb.	7.7	1.4	15.2	84
Croaker, Fresh	4 oz.	20.2	2.5	(0)	109
Cucumbers, fresh sliced (6 slices 1/8 thick)	50 gm.	.4	(0)	1.4	6

FOOD DESCRIPTION	UNIT OF MEASURE	PROTEIN Gm.	FAT Gm.	CARBOHYDRATES Gm.	CALORIES (energy)
Custard, baked	1 cup	13.1	13.4	27.8	283
Dates, fresh, dried, pitted	1 cup	3.9	1.1	134.2	505
Doughnuts, cake type (standard size)	1 pc.	2.1	6.7	16.9	136
Eggs, chicken, fresh, stored or frozen	1 med.	6.1	5.5	.3	77
Eggs, whites only (from 1 med. egg)	31 gm.	3.3	(0)	.2	15
Eggs, yolks only (from 1 med. egg)	17 gm.	2.8	5.4	.1	61
Farina, cooked	1 cup	3.1	.2	21.7	104
Fats, cooking (vegetable type)	1 Tbsp.	(0)	12.5	(0)	101
Figs, fresh (1 ½" dia.)	3 sml.	1.6	.5	22.3	90
Figs, canned in syrup (3 figs, 2 Tbsp. syrup)	114 gm.	.9	.3	34.2	129
Figs, dried (1 large 2" x 1" in size)	21 gm.	.8	.3	14.4	57
Flounder, fresh, summer or winter	4 oz.	16.9	.6	(0)	78
Frankfurters, standard size	51 gm.	7.0	10.0	1.0	124
Frogs Legs, fresh, cooked	4 oz.	18.6	.3	(0)	82
Fruit Cocktail, cand. solids and liquids	1 cup	1.0	.5	47.6	179

FOOD DESCRIPTION	UNIT OF MEASURE	PRO-TEIN Gm.	FAT Gm.	CARBO-HYDRATES Gm.	CAL-ORIES (energy)
Gelatin Dessert, ready to serve, plain	1 cup	3.8	(0)	36.3	155
Gelatin Dessert, ready, with fruit added	1 cup	3.4	.2	42.2	172
Gooseberries, fresh	1 cup	1.2	.3	14.6	59
Grapefruit, (1/2 med. 4 ½" dia.)	285 gm.	.9	.4	19.0	75
Grapefruit (1/2 lg. 5" dia.)	395 gm.	1.3	.5	26.4	104
Grapefruit, canned in syrup	1 cup	1.5	.5	47.6	181
Grapefruit, canned and sweetened	1 cup	1.3	.3	34.9	132
Grapefruit, canned and unsweetened	1 cup	1.5	.2	25.6	99
Grapefruit juice, fresh	1 cup	1.2	.2	22.6	87
Grapefruit juice, canned and sweetened	1 cup	1.3	.3	34.4	131
Grapefruit juice, canned and unsweetened	1 cup	1.2	.2	24.1	92
Grapes, fresh, American type	1 cup	1.7	1.7	17.7	84
Grapes, fresh, European type Green Thompson Seedless	1 cup	1.2	.6	25.9	102
Grape juice, commercial bottled	1 cup	1.0	(0)	46.2	170
Guavas, common type, fresh	1 med.	.7	.4	12.0	48

FOOD DESCRIPTION	UNIT OF MEASURE	PRO-TEIN Gm.	FAT Gm.	CARBO-HYDRATES Gm.	CAL-ORIES (energy)
Haddock, cooked or fried (4" x 3" x 1/2" fillet)	1 pc.	18.7	5.5	7.0	158
Halibut, cooked broiled (4" x 3" x 1/2" steak)	1 pc.	32.8	9.8	(0)	228
Heart, beef, lean	3 oz.	14.4	3.1	.6	92
Heart, calves, canned, strained, infants	1 oz.	3.8	.7	.1	23
Heart, chicken	3 oz.	17.4	6.0	1.4	134
Heart, pork	3 oz.	17.4	4.1	.3	100
Herring, Atlantic	4 oz.	20.8	14.2	(0)	217
Herring, lake	4 oz.	21.0	7.7	(0)	159
Herring, Pacific	4 oz.	18.8	2.9	(0)	106
Herring, smoked, kippered	3 oz.	18.9	11.0	(0)	180
Honey, strained	1 Tbsp.	.1	(0)	16.7	62
Honeydew melon, fresh (2" x 7" wedge)	150 gm.	.8	(0)	12.8	49
Ice cream, plain & flavored (1/7 of qt.)	81 gm.	3.2	10.1	16.7	167
Jams, marmalades, preserves	1 Tbsp.	.1	.1	14.2	55
Jellies	1 Tbsp.	(0)	(0)	13.0	50
Kale, cooked, fresh	1 cup	4.3	.7	7.9	45
Kidneys, beef	3 oz.	12.8	6.9	.8	120
Kidneys, pork	3 oz.	13.9	3.9	.7	97

FOOD DESCRIPTION	UNIT OF MEASURE	PROTEIN Gm.	FAT Gm.	CARBOHYDRATES Gm.	CALORIES (energy)
Kidneys, sheep	3 oz.	14.1	2.8	.9	89
Lamb, rib chop, cooked, without bone	3 oz.	20.0	30.0	(0)	356
Lamb shoulder roast, ckd, w/o bone	3 oz.	18.0	24.0	(0)	192
Lamb, leg roast, cooked, without bone	3 oz.	20.0	16.0	(0)	120
Lamb, canned, strained, infants, food	1 oz.	4.0	1.3	(0)	30
Lamb & Vegetable Soup, canned, strained	1 oz.	.7	.3	2.2	14
Lard	1 Tbsp.	(0)	14.0	(0)	126
Lemons (1 med. 2 3/4" x 2")	100 gm.	.6	.4	5.4	20
Lemon juice, fresh extracted	1 Tbsp.	.1	(0)	1.2	4
Lemon juice, canned & unsweetened	1 Tbsp.	.1	(0)	1.2	4
Lettuce, head, fresh (2 large or 4 small leaves)	50 gm.	.6	.1	1.4	7
Limes, (medium 2: dia. size)	68 gm.	.4	.1	6.4	19
Lime juice, fresh extracted	1 cup	1.0	(0)	20.4	58
Liver, Beef, cooked-fried	2 oz.	13.4	4.4	5.5	118
Liver, calves, broiled	3 oz.	16.2	4.2	3.4	120

FOOD DESCRIPTION	UNIT OF MEASURE	PROTEIN	FAT	CARBOHYDRATE	CALORIES
		Gm.	Gm.	Gm.	(energy)
Liver, chicken, broiled	3 oz.	18.8	3.4	2.2	320
Liver, Pork, Broiled	3 oz.	16.7	4.1	1.4	114
Liver, sheep, broiled (or Lamb)	3 oz.	17.8	3.3	2.5	116
Liverwurst, liver sausage	1 oz.	9.5	11.7	.9	150
Lobster, canned	3 oz.	15.6	1.1	.3	78
Loganberries, fresh	1 cup	1.4	.9	21.6	90
Macaroni, cooked	1 cup	7.1	.8	42.3	209
Mackeral, canned Atlantic & Pacific	3 oz.	16.4	8.4	(0)	155
Mangoes, fresh (1 med. size)	100 gm.	.9	.3	22.7	87
Margerine (vegetable table spread)	1 Tbsp.	.1	11.3	.1	101
Margarine (vegetable table spread)	1 patty	(0)	5.7	(0)	50
Milk, whole, pasteurized	1 cup	8.5	9.5	12.0	166
Milk, non-fat, (skimmed)	1 cup	8.6	.3	12.5	87
Milk, evaporated, unsweetened	1 cup	17.6	19.9	24.9	346
Milk, condensed & sweetened	1 cup	24.8	25.7	167.7	981
Milk, Malted beverage	1 cup	12.4	21.9	31.9	281
Milk, goat, fresh, fluid	1 cup	8.1	9.8	9.8	164

FOOD DESCRIPTION	UNIT OF MEASURE	PRO-TEIN Gm.	FAT Gm.	CARBO-HYDRATES Gm.	CAL-ORIES (energy)
Molasses, light, first extraction	1 Tbsp.	(0)	(0)	13.0	50
Molasses, blackstrap, 3rd extraction	1 Tbsp.	(0)	(0)	11.0	43
Molasses, Barbados	1 Tbsp.	(0)	(0)	14.0	54
Mushrooms, canned, solids and liquids	1 cup	3.4	.5	9.0	28
Noodles, containing egg, cooked	1 cup	3.5	1.0	20.5	107
Oat cereal, ready to eat type	1 cup	3.6	1.8	17.6	100
Oatmeal (rolled oats) cooked	1 cup	5.4	2.8	26.0	148
Oils, salad or dressing	1 Tbsp.	(0)	14.0	(0)	124
Okra, cooked (8 pods, 3" lg x 5.8" dia.)	85 gm.	1.5	.2	6.3	28
Olives, pickled green	10 med.	.8	7.4	2.2	72
Olives, ripe	10 med.	1.0	11.6	1.4	106
Onions, mature, raw (1 med. 2 1/2" dia.)	1 med.	1.5	.2	11.3	49
Onions, cooked, whole	1 cup	2.1	.4	18.3	79
Oranges, fresh, lge. (3 3/8" dia.)	1 lg.	2.1	.5	26.2	106
Oranges, fresh, med. (3" dia.)	1 med.	1.4	.3	17.4	70

FOOD DESCRIPTION	UNIT OF MEASURE	PROTEIN Gm.	FAT Gm.	CARBOHYDRATES Gm.	CALORIES (energy)
Oranges, fresh, small, (2 1/2" dia.)	1 sm.	1.0	.2	12.1	49
Orange juice, fresh extracted	1 cup	2.0	.5	27.1	108
Orange juice, canned, unsweetened	1 cup	2.0	.5	27.3	109
Orange juice, canned, sweetened	1 cup	1.5	.5	34.9	135
Orange juice, canned, concentrated, frozen	6 fl. oz.	5.5	1.4	74.9	300
Oysters, raw, meat only	1 cup	23.5	5.0	13.4	200
Oysters, Stew (1 pt. Oysters, 3 pts. milk)	1 cup	12.2	12.4	12.2	209
Oyster Stew (1 pt. Oysters, 1 pt. milk)	1 cup	16.6	13.2	14.2	244
Pancakes, griddlecakes, baked 4" dia.	1 cake	1.8	2.5	7.2	59
Pancakes, buckwheat, baked (4" dia.)	1 cake	1.6	2.3	5.6	47
Papaya, fresh, (1/2" cubes)	1 cup	1.1	.2	18.2	71
Parsley, common type, fresh, chopped	1 Tbsp.	.1	(0)	.3	1
Parsnips, cooked	1 cup	1.6	.8	21.5	94
Peaches, fresh, raw, medium size	1 pc.	.5	.1	12.0	46
Peaches, canned, water packed	1 cup	1.2	.2	16.6	66

FOOD DESCRIPTION	UNIT OF MEASURE	PROTEIN Gm.	FAT Gm.	CARBO-HYDRATES Gm.	CALORIES (energy)
Peaches, canned, syrup packed	1 cup	1.0	.3	46.6	174
Peaches, frozen	4 oz.	.5	.1	22.9	89
Peaches, fresh, cooked, sugar added	1 cup	2.4	.6	95.5	366
Peanuts, Virginia type roasted, shelled	1 cup	38.7	63.6	34.0	805
Peanut Butter	1 Tbsp.	4.2	7.6	3.4	92
Pears, fresh, raw, (3" x 2½" dia.)	1 med.	1.1	.6	23.9	95
Pears, canned, water packed	1 cup	.7	.2	19.8	75
Pears, canned, syrup packed	1 cup	.5	.3	47.1	174
Peas, green, fresh, cooked	1 cup	7.8	.6	19.4	111
Peas, green, canned, drained	1 cup	7.2	1.0	27.5	145
Pea soup, condensed	11 oz.	16.2	5.0	63.6	357
Pea soup, ready to serve	1 cup	6.4	2.0	25.0	141
Pecans, halves of meat	1 cup	10.2	78.8	14.0	752
Pecans, chopped	1 Tbsp.	.7	5.5	1.0	52
Peppers, green, fresh, med. size	1 med.	.8	.1	3.6	16
Persimmons, Japanese of Kaki, fresh	1 med.	1.0	.5	24.2	95

FOOD DESCRIPTION	UNIT OF MEASURE	PRO-TEIN Gm.	FAT Gm.	CARBO-HYDRATES Gm.	CAL-ORIES (energy)
Pickles, dill, cucumber (4" lg x 2 1/4" dia.)	1 large	.9	.3	2.8	15
Pickles, sour, mixed (4" lg x 1 3/4" dia.)	1 large	.7	.3	3.0	15
Pickles, sweet, mixed (2 3/4" lg x 3/4" dia.)	1 med.	.2	.1	5.3	22
Pimentos, canned (1 med. size)	38 gm.	.3	.2	2.2	10
Pineapple, fresh (3 1/2" dia. x 3/4" thick)	1 slice	.3	.2	11.5	44
Pineapple, canned, crushed, in syrup	1 cup	1.0	.3	54.9	204
Pineapple, canned, sliced, in syrup	1 sl.	.5	.1	25.7	95
Pineapple, canned and frozen	4 oz.	.5	.2	25.2	97
Pineapple, juice, canned	1 cup	.7	.2	32.4	121
Plums, fresh, all types, (incl. prunes)	1 cup	1.3	.4	23.9	94
Plums, canned, in syrup	1 cup	1.0	.2	50.2	186
Popcorn, popped	1 cup	1.8	.7	10.7	54
Pork, ham without bone	3 oz.	20.0	28.0	(0)	338
Pork, loin or chops, without bone	3 oz.	20.0	22.0	(0)	284
Pork, ham, cured, smoked, no bone	3 oz.	20.0	28.0	.3	339

FOOD DESCRIPTION	UNIT OF MEASURE	PROTEIN Gm.	FAT Gm.	CARBO-HYDRATES Gm.	CALORIES (energy)
Pork, luncheon meat, boiled	2 oz.	12.9	12.9	(0)	172
Pork, luncheon meat, canned, spiced	2 oz.	8.4	13.8	.9	164
Pork, sausage, links or bulk	4 oz.	12.2	50.8	(0)	510
Potatoes, baked (med. 2 1/2" dia.)	128 gm.	2.4	.1	22.3	97
Potatoes, boiled, (med. 2 1/2" dia.)	150 gm.	2.8	.1	27.1	118
Potatoes, French-fried (2" x 1/2" x 1/2")	8 pcs.	2.2	7.6	20.8	157
Potatoes, hash-browned	1 cup	6.4	22.8	62.2	470
Potatoes, mashed, milk added	1 cup	4.3	1.4	33.2	159
Potatoes, mashed, milk & butter added	1 cup	4.1	11.7	31.0	240
Potatoes, steamed or pressure cooked	1 med.	2.5	.1	24.1	105
Potatoes, canned, solids & liquid	1 cup	4.2	(0)	32.8	144
Potato chips (med. wafers 2" dia.)	10 pcs.	1.3	7.4	9.8	108
Pretzels, small sticks	5 sml.	.4	.2	3.7	18
Prunes, dried, unsulphured, uncooked	4 lg.	.8	.2	24.8	94
Prunes, cooked, no sugar	1 cup	2.7	.7	81.8	310
Prunes, cooked, sugar added	1 cup	2.9	.6	126.6	483

FOOD DESCRIPTION	UNIT OF MEASURE	PROTEINS Gm.	FAT Gm.	CARBOHYDRATES Gm.	CALORIES (energy)
Prune juice, canned	1 cup	1.0	(0)	46.3	170
Prune Whip (standard recipe)	1 cup	3.8	.4	50.1	200
Pumpkin, canned	1 cup	2.3	.7	18.0	76
Radishes, fresh (4 small)	40 gm.	.2	(0)	.8	4
Raisins, dried, unsulphured	1 Tbsp.	.2	(0)	7.1	26
Raspberries, red, fresh	1 cup	1.5	.3	17.0	70
Raspberries, red frozen	3 oz.	.7	.3	21.0	84
Rhubarb, fresh, diced	1 cup	.6	.1	4.6	19
Rhubarb, cooked, sugar added	1 cup	1.8	.3	97.9	383
Rice, Brown, raw	1 cup	15.6	3.5	161.6	748
Rice, converted, cooked	1 cup	4.2	.2	44.7	204
Rice, white or milled, cooked	1 cup	4.2	.2	44.0	201
Rice, precooked, dry	1 cup	9.7	.2	91.6	420
Rice flakes	1 cup	1.8	.2	26.3	118
Rice, puffed	1 cup	.8	.1	12.3	55
Rolls, plain or pan rolls (med. size)	1 roll	3.4	2.1	20.9	118
Rolls, sweet (med. size)	1 roll	4.7	4.3	29.6	178
Rutabagas, cooked	1 cup	1.2	.2	11.6	50

FOOD DESCRIPTION	UNIT OF MEASURE	PROTEINS Gm.	FAT Gm.	CARBO-HYDRATES Gm.	CALORIES (energy)
Salad dressing (mayonnaise type)	1 Tbsp.	.2	5.5	2.1	58
Salad dressing (French type)	1 Tbsp.	.1	5.3	3.0	59
Salad Dressing, homecooked, boiled	1 Tbsp.	.8	1.7	2.6	28
Salad Dressing (regular mayonnaise)	1 Tbsp.	.2	10.1	.4	92
Salmon, Pacific, broiled or baked (4" x 3" x 1/2")	1 pc.	33.6	6.7	.2	204
Salmon, canned, (most brands)	3 oz.	17.9	7.1	(0)	140
Sardines, Atlantic type, in oil	3 oz.	17.9	23.0	.9	288
Sardines, Pacific type, natural pack	3 oz.	15.1	11.5	.6	171
Sardines, Pacific type, in tomato sauce	3 oz.	15.1	12.6	1.4	184
Sauerkraut, canned, drained	1 cup	2.1	.4	6.6	32
Sausage, bologna (1" x 2 3/4 dia.)	211 gm.	31.2	33.5	7.6	467
Sausage, frankfurter (1 standard size)	51 gm.	7.0	10.0	1.0	124
Sausage, liver, liverwurst	2 oz.	9.5	11.7	.9	150
Sausage, Vienna, canned	4 oz.	17.9	18.6	(0)	244
Scallops, fresh	4 oz.	16.8	.1	3.9	89

FOOD DESCRIPTION	UNIT OF MEASURE	PROTEIN Gm.	FAT Gm.	CARBO-HYDRATES Gm.	CALORIES (energy)
Shad or American Shad	4 oz.	21.2	11.1	(0)	191
Sherbert, all flavors	1/2 cup	1.4	(0)	28.8	118
Shortbread (2 squares 1 3/4" square)	2 pcs.	1.1	3.9	10.3	81
Shrimp, canned, dry pack	3 oz.	22.8	1.2	(0)	108
Shrimp, canned wet pack	3 oz.	15.9	.8	.3	76
Syrup, table blends, (chiefly corn)	1 Tbsp.	(0)	(0)	14.8	57
Soups, bean, canned, condensed	11 oz.	21.5	12.8	73.6	481
Soups, bean, canned, ready to serve	1 cup	8.5	5.0	29.5	191
Soups, beef, canned, condensed	11 oz.	15.0	8.4	27.8	248
Soups, beef, canned, ready to serve	1 cup	6.0	3.5	11.0	100
Soups, bouillon broth, condensed, canned	11 oz.	6.0	(0)	(0)	26
Soups, bouillon broth, ready to serve	1 cup	2.0	(0)	(0)	9
Soups, chicken, condensed, canned	11 oz.	8.4	5.9	24.6	187
Soups, chicken, ready to serve, canned	1 cup	3.5	2.5	9.5	75
Soups, clam chowder, condensed, canned	11 oz.	10.9	5.9	30.2	210

FOOD DESCRIPTION	UNIT OF MEASURE	PROTEIN	FAT	CARBOHYDRATE	CALORIES
		Gm.	Gm.	Gm.	(energy)
Soups, clam chowder, ready to serve	1 cup	4.6	2.3	12.5	86
Soups, cream soups, all kinds, condensed	11 oz.	6.9	16.2	29.6	279
Soups, cream soups, ready to serve	1 cup	7.1	11.7	18.4	201
Soups, noodle or barley, condensed, canned	11 oz.	15.3	10.9	32.4	291
Soups, noodle or barley, ready to serve	1 cup	6.0	4.5	13.0	117
Soups, pea, condensed, canned	11 oz.	16.2	5.0	63.6	357
Soups, pea, ready to serve, canned	1 cup	6.4	2.0	25.0	141
Soups, tomato, condensed, canned	11 oz.	5.6	5.6	45.5	230
Soups, tomato, ready to serve, canned	1 cup	2.2	2.2	17.9	90
Soups, vegetable, condensed, canned	11 oz.	10.3	4.4	35.9	203
Soybean sprouts, fresh	1 cup	6.6	1.5	5.7	49
Spaghetti, cooked	1 cup	7.4	.9	44.1	218
Spinach, cooked, canned	1 cup	5.6	1.1	6.5	46
Squash, summer, cooked, diced	1 cup	1.3	.2	8.2	34
Squash, winter, cooked, mashed	1 cup	3.9	.8	22.6	97
Strawberries, fresh	1 cup	1.2	.7	12.4	54

FOOD DESCRIPTION	UNIT OF MEASURE	PRO-TEIN	FAT	CARBO-HYDRATES	CAL-ORIES
		Gm.	Gm.	Gm.	(energy)
Strawberries, frozen	3 oz.	.5	.3	22.6	90
Sugars, granulated, cane or beet	1 Tbsp.	(0)	(0)	12.4	48
Sugars, granulated, cane or beet	1 tsp.	(0)	(0)	4.2	16
Sugars, powdered	1 Tbsp.	(0)	(0)	8.0	31
Sugars, brown	1 Tbsp.	(0)	(0)	13.1	51
Sugars, maple (piece 1 3/4" x 1 1/4" x 1/2")	30 gm.	(0)	(0)	27.0	104
Sweet potatoes (5" x 2 1/2" dia.) baked	120 gm.	2.6	1.1	41.3	183
Sweet potatoes, (5" x 1/2" dia.) boiled	205 gm.	3.7	1.4	57.2	252
Sweet potatoes, candied (3 1/2" x 2 1/4") sm.	175 gm.	2.6	6.3	63.4	314
Swordfish, broiled (steak 3" x 3" x 1/2")	125 gm.	34.2	8.5	(0)	223
Tangerines, medium size (2 1/2" dia.)	114 gm.	.6	.2	8.8	35
Tangerine juice, fresh extracted	1 cup	2.2	.7	22.6	95
Tangerine juice, canned, unsweetened	1 cup	2.2	.7	22.6	95
Tomatoes, fresh (med. 2" x 2 1/2" dia.)	150 gm.	1.5	.4	6.0	30
Tomatoes, canned, cooked	1 cup	2.4	.5	9.4	46

FOOD DESCRIPTION	UNIT OF MEASURE	PROTEIN Gm.	FAT Gm.	CARBO-HYDRATES Gm.	CALORIES (energy)
Tomato juice, canned	1 cup	2.4	.5	10.4	50
Tomato catsup	1 Tbsp.	.3	.1	4.2	17
Tomato Puree, canned	1 cup	4.5	1.2	17.9	90
Tongue, beef, med. fat	4 oz.	18.6	17.0	.5	235
Tortillas, (med. 5" dia.)	20 gm.	1.2	.6	9.7	50
Tuna fish, canned	3 oz.	24.7	7.0	(0)	169
Turkey, med. fat cooked	4 oz.	22.8	22.9	(0)	304
Turnips, cooked, diced	1 cup	1.2	.3	9.3	42
Turnip greens, boiled	1 cup	4.2	.6	7.8	43
Veal cutlet, cooked without bone	3 oz.	24.0	9.0	(0)	183
Veal, shoulder roast, without bone	3 oz.	24.0	10.0	(0)	193
Veal, stew meat, cooked, without bone	3 oz.	21.0	18.0	(0)	252
Vinegar, all types	1 Tbsp.	(0)	(0)	.8	2
Waffles (4 1/2" x 5 5/8" x 1/2")	1 pc.	7.0	8.0	28.4	216
Walnuts, Persian or English, halves	1 cup	15.0	64.4	15.6	654
Watermelon (1/16th melon, 16" x 10")	925 gm.	2.1	.9	29.4	120
Wheat bran flakes	1 cup	3.8	.6	28.1	125

FOOD DESCRIPTION	UNIT OF MEASURE	PROTEIN	FAT	CARBO-HYDRATES	CALORIES
		Gm.	Gm.	Gm.	(energy)
Wheat germ, stirred	1 cup	17.1	6.8	33.7	246
Wheat, puffed, breakfast cereal	1 cup	1.3	.2	9.6	43
Wheat, rolled, cooked	1 cup	5.2	.9	39.9	177
Wheat, shredded, (4" x 2 1/4" biscuit)	1 bisc.	2.9	.7	22.7	102
Wild Rice, parched, raw	1 cup	23.0	1.1	122.7	593
Yeast, compressed, bakers	1 oz.	3.0	.1	3.7	24
Yeast, dried, brewer's yeast	1 Tbsp.	3.0	.1	3.0	22

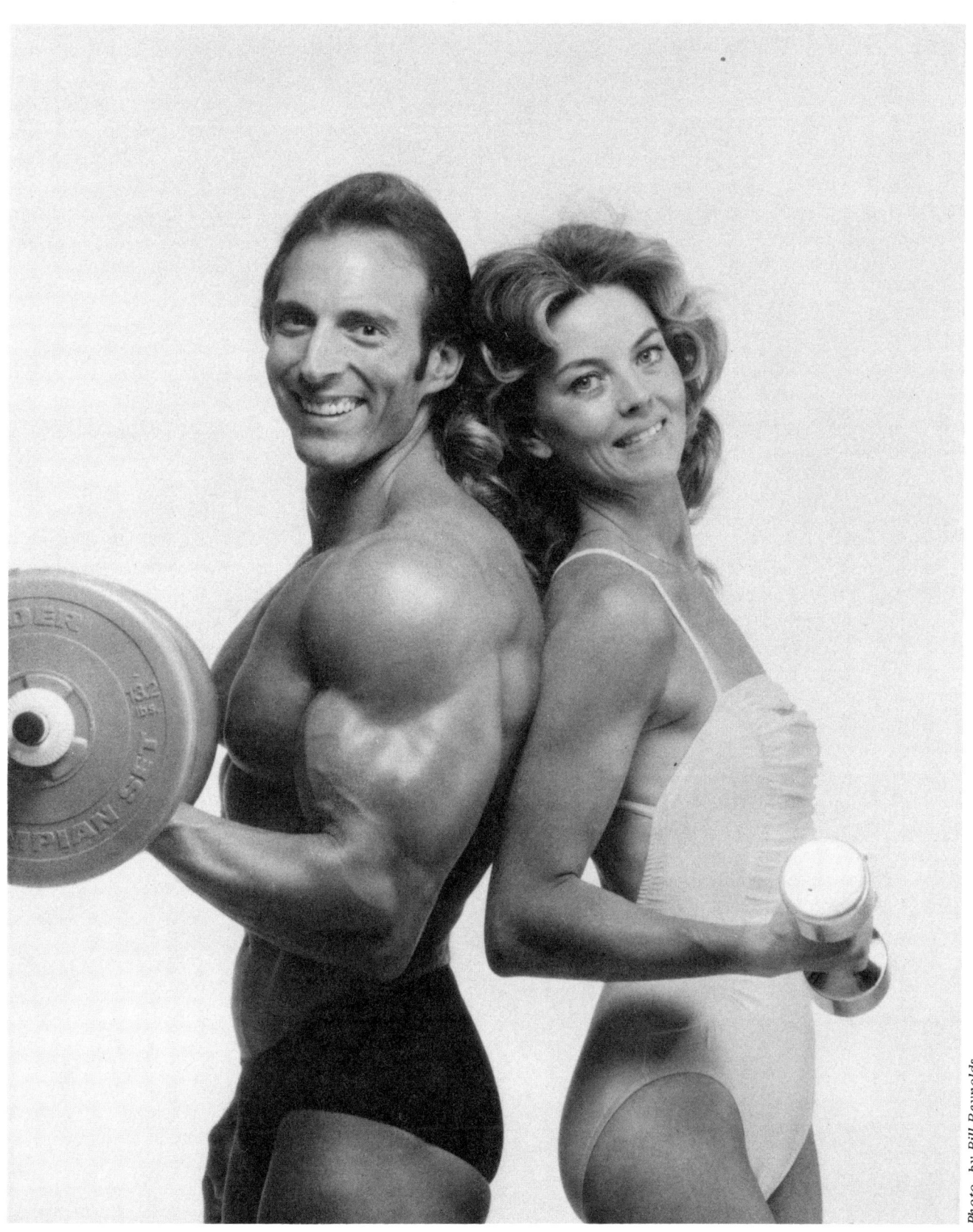

PAT AND VICKI NEVE